DEMONSTRATING YOUR CLINICAL COMPETENCE IN DEPRESSION, DEMENTIA, ALCOHOLISM, PALLIATIVE CARE AND OSTEOPOROSIS

Jane Higgs
Gill Wakley
Ruth Chambers
and
Clare Gerada

RADCLIFFE PUBLISHING
Oxford • Seattle

Radcliffe Publishing Ltd
18 Marcham Road
Abingdon
Oxon OX14 1AA
United Kingdom

www.radcliffe-oxford.com
Electronic catalogue and worldwide online ordering facility.

British Library Cataloguing in Publication Data

A catalogue record for this book is available from the British Library.

ISBN 1 85775 744 0

Typeset by Advance Typesetting Ltd, Oxford
Printed and bound by TJ International Ltd, Padstow, Cornwall

Contents

Preface

The Nursing and Midwifery Council requires nurses to maintain a professional portfolio.[1] The onus is on individual nurses to decide how they will collect and keep the information that will show that they are clinically competent and that they have taken on board the concept of lifelong learning. Nurses themselves need to decide the nature of the information they collect and retain, in order to have their everyday roles and responsibilities most accurately represented. The National Prescribing Centre[2] along with the Department of Health and professional organisations also requires nurse prescribers to maintain their competency in prescribing.

This book is one of a series that will guide you as a nurse though the process, giving you examples and ideas as to how to document your learning, competence, performance or standards of service delivery. Chapter 1 explains the link between your personal development plans, professional portfolio and individual performance reviews. Learning and service improvements that are integral to your personal development plan are central to the evidence you include in your portfolio. The stages of the evidence cycle that we suggest are reproduced from the *Good Appraisal Toolkit*[3] emphasising the importance of documenting evidence from your learning and practice in your professional portfolio.

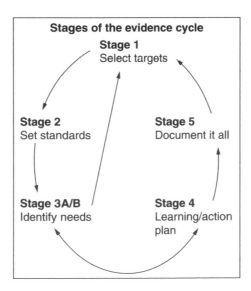

Stage 1 is about setting targets or aspirations for good practice. Stage 2 encourages you, as a nurse, to set standards for the outcomes of what you plan to learn more about, or outcomes relating to you providing a good service in your practice.

Chapter 2 describes a variety of methods to help you to address Stage 3 of the cycle of evidence, to find out what it is you need to learn about or what gaps there are in the way you deliver care as an individual or as a team. This chapter includes a wide variety of methods nurses might use in their everyday work to identify and document these needs. One of the main drivers for striving to improve practice is to benefit individual patients. So it makes sense that we have emphasised the importance of obtaining feedback from patients in this chapter in relation to identifying your learning and service development needs.

Best practice in addressing the giving of informed consent by patients, maintaining confidentiality of patient information and organising responsive complaints processes are all common components of good quality healthcare. Chapter 3 covers these aspects in depth and provides the first example of cycles of evidence for you to consider adopting or adapting for your own circumstances.

The rest of the book consists of five clinically based chapters that mainly span key topics in meeting the General Medical Services (GMS) quality framework. Attention to these areas can ensure that achieving quality points for the practice also achieves positive clinical outcomes for the patients. Some of the quality indicators are generic to various clinical areas such as smoking status, smoking cessation advice and influenza immunisation, and they obviously overlap. Others such as good record keeping, a consistent approach to maintaining disease registers, medicines management and education/appraisal of staff should underpin all the clinical areas. As we cover the five clinical topics in this book in Chapters 4 to 8, we point out what quality points are available in that clinical area. Other books in the series also include clinical topics within the scope of the GMS quality framework – so it will be useful for you to read them too (e.g. coronary heart disease, stroke and epilepsy are included in: Higgs J, Wakley G, Chambers R and Ellis S (2004) *Demonstrating Your Clinical Competence in Cardiovascular and Neurological Conditions*. Radcliffe Publishing, Oxford).

The first part of each clinical chapter covers key issues that are likely to crop up in typical clinical scenarios. The second part of each chapter gives examples of cycles of evidence in a similar format to those in Chapter 3.

Overall, you will probably want to choose three or four cycles of evidence each year. You might choose one or two from Chapter 3 and the rest from clinical areas such as those covered by Chapters 4 to 8. You might like this way of learning and service development so much that you build up a bigger bank of evidence, taking one cycle from each chapter in the same year. Whatever your approach, you will want to keep your cycles of evidence as short and simple as possible, so that the documentation itself is a by-product of the learning and action plans you undertake to improve the service you provide, and does not dominate your time and effort at work.

Other books in the series are based on the same format of the five stages in the cycle of evidence. Book 1 helps nurses and other health professionals to demonstrate that they are competent teachers or trainers, and Books 2, 3 and 4 set out key information and examples of evidence for a wide variety of clinical areas for nurses and other healthcare practitioners.

This approach and style of learning will take a bit of getting used to for many nurses. Until recently, most nurses did not reflect on what they learnt or whether they applied it in practice. They did not protect time for learning and reflection among their everyday responsibilities, or target their time and effort on priority topics. Times are changing, and with the introduction of personal development plans and individual performance reviews, nurses are realising that they must take a more professional approach to learning and document their standards of competence, performance and service delivery. This book helps them to do just that.

Please note that resources to support this book are provided at http:// health.mattersonline.net.

References

1 www.nmc-uk.org (accessed 25 April 2005)

2 www.npc.co.uk (accessed 25 April 2005)

3 Chambers R, Tavabie A, Mohanna K and Wakley G (2004) *The Good Appraisal Toolkit for Primary Care*. Radcliffe Publishing, Oxford.

About the authors

Jane Higgs has worked in primary care predominantly in district nursing and in practice nursing. She trained as a community practice educator (CPE) and is currently clinical practice development nurse for district nurses, health visitors and practice nurses, supporting health professionals to improve their clinical practice through benchmarking, clinical supervision and evidence-based guidelines and by providing advice and training support. She has been involved in developing clinical practice benchmarks and core competency frameworks regionally. She has developed various educational initiatives and training activities and is also the nurse prescribing lead for a primary care trust in the northwest of England.

Gill Wakley started in general practice but transferred to community medicine shortly afterwards and then into public health. A desire for increased contact with patients caused a move back into general practice. She has been heavily involved in learning and teaching throughout her career. She was in a training general practice, became an instructing doctor and a regional assessor in family planning, and was until recently a senior clinical lecturer with the Primary Care Department at Keele University. Like Ruth, she has run all types of educational initiatives and activities. A visiting professor at Staffordshire University, she now works as a freelance GP, writer and lecturer.

Ruth Chambers has been a general practitioner (GP) for more than 20 years and is currently the head of the Stoke-on-Trent Teaching Primary Care Trust programme and professor of primary care development at Staffordshire University. Ruth has worked with the Royal College of General Practitioners (RCGP) to enable GPs to gather evidence about their learning and standards of practice while striving to be excellent GPs. Ruth has co-authored a series of books with Gill, designed to help readers draw up their own personal development plan or workplace learning plans around key clinical topics.

Clare Gerada has been a GP in a South London practice for 14 years and previously trained as a psychiatrist at the Maudsley Hospital. She has a special interest in drug misuse and leads the RCGP's drug misuse training programme. She has worked in the Department of Health in various guises for a number of years and is currently Director of Primary Care for the Clinical Governance Support Team. She has published widely on a number of topics related to drug and alcohol problems, primary care and clinical governance. She led the RCGP development of the frameworks for general practitioners with special interests.

1

Making the link: personal development plans, post-registration education and practice (PREP) and portfolios

The process of lifelong learning

The professional regulatory body for nursing, the Nursing and Midwifery Council (NMC), has stated within the Professional Code of Conduct (2002) that all registered nurses must maintain their professional knowledge and competence.[1] The code states 'you should take part regularly in learning activities that develop your competence and performance'. This means that learning should be lifelong and encompass continuing professional development (CPD). The formal requirements for nurses to re-register state that nurses must meet the post-registration education and practice standards (PREP). This includes completion of 750 hours in practice during the five years prior to renewal of registration, together with evidence that the nurse has met the professional standards for CPD. This standard comprises a minimum of five days' (or 35 hours') learning activity relevant to the nurse's clinical practice in the three years prior to renewal of professional registration.[2] This requirement is seen as minimal by many nurses who would profess to undertake much more CPD than this in order to keep themselves abreast of current changes in practice. However, many nurses pay little attention to the recording of their CPD activity. This chapter will help you to identify a suitable format for recording learning that occurs in both clinical and educational settings.

Learning involves many steps. It includes the acquisition of information, its retention, the ability to retrieve the information when needed and how to use that information for best practice. Demonstrating your learning involves being able to show the steps you have taken. CPD takes time. It makes sense to utilise the time spent by overlapping learning undertaken to meet your personal and professional needs with that required for the performance of your role in the health service.

All nurses are required to maintain a personal professional portfolio of their learning activity. This is essential to maintain registration with the NMC.[2] Many nurses have drawn up a personal development plan (PDP) that is agreed with their line manager. Some nurses have constructed their PDP in a systematic way and identified the priorities within it, or gathered evidence to demonstrate that what they learnt about was subsequently applied in practice. The NMC does not have a uniform approach to the style of a PDP. Some nurse tutors or managers are content to see that a plan has been drawn up, while others encourage the nurse to develop a systematic approach to identifying and addressing their learning and service needs, in order of importance or urgency.

The new emphasis on lifelong learning for nurses has given the PDP a higher profile. Nurse educationalists view a PDP as a tool to encourage nurses to plan their own learning activities. Managers may view it as a tool that allows quality assurance of the nurse's performance. Nurses, striving to improve the quality of the care that they deliver to patients, may want to use a PDP to guide them on their way, perhaps towards post-registration awards or towards gaining promotion opportunities.

Your personal development plan

Your PDP will be an integral part of your annual appraisal (sometimes referred to as an individual performance review) and your portfolio that is required by the NMC to demonstrate your fitness to practise as a nurse.

Your initial plan should:

- identify your gaps or weaknesses in knowledge, skills or attitudes
- specify topics for learning as a result of changes: in your role, responsibilities, the organisation in which you work
- link into the learning needs of others in your workplace or team of colleagues
- tie in with the service development priorities of your practice, the primary care organisation (PCO), hospital trust or the NHS as a whole
- describe how you identified your learning needs
- set your learning needs and associated goals in order of importance and urgency
- justify your selection of learning goals
- describe how you will achieve your goals and over what time period
- describe how you will evaluate learning outcomes.[3]

Each year you will continue to revise your personal development plan to support the development review process of *The NHS Knowledge and Skills Framework (NHS KSF)*.[4] It should demonstrate how you carried out your learning and evaluation plans, show that you have learnt what you set out to do (or why it was modified) and how you applied your new learning in practice. In addition, you will find that you have new priorities and fresh learning needs as circumstances change.

The main task is to capture what you have learnt, in a way that suits you. Then you can look back at what you have done and:

- reflect on it later, to decide to learn more, or to make changes as a result, and identify further needs
- demonstrate to others that you are fit to practise or work through:
  - what you have done
  - what you have learnt

- – what changes you have made as a result
- – the standards of work you have achieved and are maintaining
- – how you monitor your performance at work
- use it to show how your personal learning fits in with the requirements of your practice or the NHS, and other people's personal and professional development plans.

Incorporate all the evidence of your learning into your personal professional profile (PPP). Evidence from this document will be needed if you are asked to take part in the NMC audit, which is designed to ensure that all nurses are complying with the PREP standard. It is up to you how you keep this record of your learning. Examples are:

- *an ongoing learning journal* in which you draw up and describe your plan, record how you determined your needs and prioritised them, report why you attended particular educational meetings or courses and what you got out of them as well as the continuing cycle of review, making changes and evaluating them
- *an A4 file* with lots of plastic sleeves into which you build up a systematic record of your educational activities in line with your plan
- *a box*: chuck in everything to do with your learning plan as you do it and sort it out into a sensible order every few months with a good review once a year.

Using portfolios for appraisal/individual performance review, KSF and PREP

Appraisal is widely accepted in the NHS as a formative process that should be concerned with the professional development and personal fulfilment of the individual, leading to an improvement in their performance at work. It is a formal structured opportunity whereby the person being appraised has the opportunity to reflect on their work and to consider how their effectiveness might be improved. This positive interpretation of the appraisal process supports the delivery of high-quality patient care and drive to improve clinical standards. Appraisal has been in place in industry, commerce and public sectors for decades. In the NHS, nurses and other health professionals, managers and administrative staff are now all expected to undergo annual appraisals.

Nurses working in the health service should receive an appraisal or individual performance review at least once a year. This appraisal should include two main functions. Firstly there should be an assessment of fitness to practise in the current role, and secondly there should be a review of the CPD that has taken place and that is needed for the future. This should focus on the needs of the individual together with the needs of the organisation for which the nurse works.

Details of how annual appraisals are structured will vary from one organisation to another, but the educational principles remain the same. The aims are to give nurses an opportunity to discuss and receive regular feedback on their previous and continuing performance and identify education and development needs.

With the introduction of the Agenda for Change Knowledge and Skills Framework (KSF),[4] nurses may find their appraisal incorporated into the KSF development review process, which has been designed to identify the knowledge and skills that individuals need to apply in their post; to help guide their development; to provide a fair and objective framework to base review and development of all staff; and to provide the basis of pay progression in the service. The main purpose of the development review is to look at the way an individual member of staff is developing in relation to the duties and responsibilities of their post, their application of knowledge and skills and the consequent development needs. Your portfolio will be required as evidence for this development review.

In 1995, the United Kingdom Central Council (UKCC) introduced the need to demonstrate that you have undertaken meaningful learning activities, directly related to your nursing role. As the superseding professional body, the NMC has maintained this PREP requirement. When you apply to renew your registration as a nurse every three years, you are required to sign a Notification of Practice form that includes a declaration that you have met the PREP requirements. This means that your employer may be at liberty to ask to see your personal professional profile that will show the learning activities undertaken and how these have influenced your work. The term portfolio and profile tend to be used synonymously in nursing. A helpful view on distinguishing between the two terms has been given by Rosslyn Brown who views the portfolio as encompassing the development of the individual as a whole (including both personal and professional perspectives), whereas the profile provides a more focused approach to the professional development and may be produced for a more clearly defined audience.[5]

The English National Board (ENB) stipulated that portfolios should be incorporated into pre-registration nursing programmes in 1997.[6] This demonstrates that portfolios are designated as part of the culture of nursing. They should not be viewed simply as a tool for assessing outcomes of courses, but as meaningful documents that provide firm evidence of an individual's journey and progression within nursing. You do not need to set out your portfolio in any specific format. In fact, one of the benefits of using a portfolio is that it allows you to be creative and to produce evidence about your practice in a way that reflects your individual style. However, there are certain elements that should be included. Quinn suggests six main areas:[7]

- factual information e.g. qualifications, job description, etc
- self-evaluation of professional performance
- action plans/PDP
- documentation of any formal learning undertaken, such as courses attended, etc
- documentation of informal learning, such as reading journal articles that have altered your practice by providing a firm evidence base to follow
- documentation of hours worked between registration periods. This may be particularly important if you do not have a regular contract of employment.[7]

A portfolio will provide evidence that you have complied with the NMC Professional Code of Conduct (2002). This clearly states that your professional knowledge must be maintained in the ways given in Box 1.1.

Box 1.1: Nursing and Midwifery Council requirements for maintaining professional knowledge

- You must keep your knowledge and skills up to date throughout your working life. In particular, you should take part regularly in learning activities that develop your confidence and performance.
- To practise competently, you must possess the knowledge, skills and abilities required for lawful, safe and effective practice without direct supervision. You must acknowledge the limits of your professional competence and only undertake practice and accept responsibilities for those activities in which you are competent.
- If an aspect of practice is beyond your level of competence or outside your area of registration, you must obtain help and supervision from a competent practitioner until you and your employer consider that you have acquired the requisite knowledge and skill.
- You have a duty to facilitate students of nursing and midwifery and others to develop their competence.
- You have a responsibility to deliver care based on current evidence, best practice and, where applicable, validated research when it is available.

Reproduced from: Nursing and Midwifery Council (2002) *Code of Professional Conduct*. Nursing and Midwifery Council, London[1]

Lifelong learning is a concept that is advocated by the NMC in order to develop professional knowledge and competence in order to improve patient care.[8] Lifelong learning can be structured to ensure that learning is meaningful and relevant to your current role. The best way to do this is to incorporate a PDP as a central part of your portfolio. It provides a framework to highlight your learning needs and demonstrates self-awareness and organisation of prioritised learning. Ideally, the PDP should arise from your individual performance review, as this will have utilised both subjective and objective assessments to highlight your developmental needs.

Demonstrating the standards of your practice

The NMC sets out standards that must be met as part of the duties and responsibilities of nurses in the Professional Code of Conduct.[1] These clauses within the code have been drawn up to create expectations for the public relating to the behaviour that they can expect from nurses, and to create a uniform standard of behaviour with which all nurses must comply. A good portfolio should reflect these standards of care wherever possible. For example, confidential information should be protected, so that if your portfolio includes reflective writing there should be no way of identifying specific patients within this. The clauses within the Code of Conduct are shared values from all the UK healthcare regulatory bodies. Box 1.2 lists the requirements within the code.

Box 1.2:   Clauses to consider when creating a portfolio which relates to clinical care

In caring for patients and clients, you must:

- respect the patient or client as an individual
- obtain consent before you give any treatment or care
- protect confidential information
- co-operate with others in the team
- maintain your professional knowledge and competence
- be trustworthy
- act to identify and minimise risk to patients and clients.

Reproduced from: Nursing and Midwifery Council (2002) *Code of Professional Conduct*. Nursing and Midwifery Council, London[1]

In order to demonstrate that your clinical practice upholds these professional standards you will need to include evidence within your portfolio. The evidence cycle shown in Figure 1.1 provides a comprehensive model for demonstrating your standards of practice and how you seek to improve them. The stages of the evidence cycle are common to all the various areas of expertise considered in this book and will be followed in each chapter.

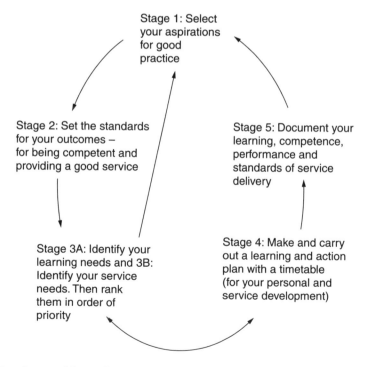

Figure 1.1:   Stages of the evidence cycle.

Although the five stages are shown in sequence here, in practice you would expect to move backwards and forwards from stage to stage, because of new information or a modification of your earlier ideas. New information might accrue when research is published which affects your clinical behaviour or standards, or a critical incident or patient complaint might occur which causes you and others to think anew about your standards or the way that services are delivered. The arrows in Figure 1.1 show that you might reset your target or aspirations for good practice, having undertaken exercises to identify what you need to learn or determine whether there are gaps in service delivery.

We suggest that you demonstrate your competence in focused areas of your day-to-day work by completing several cycles of evidence drawn from a variety of clinical or other areas each year.

As you start to collate information about this five-stage cycle, discuss any problems about the standards of care or services you are looking at, with colleagues, experts in this area, tutors, etc. You want to develop a wide range and depth of evidence so that you can show that you are competent in your day-to-day general work as well as for any special areas of expertise.

Professional competence is the first area of concern to employers and the public. You should be able to demonstrate that you can maintain a satisfactory standard of clinical care most of the time in your everyday work. Some of the time you will be brilliant, of course! Celebrate those moments. On other occasions, you or others around you will be critical of your performance and feel that you could have done much better. Reflect on those episodes to learn from them.

Stage 1: Select your aspirations for good practice

By adopting or adapting descriptions of what an 'excellent' nurse should be aiming for, you are defining the standards of practice for which you, as an individual nurse, should be aiming. You may find it easier to define your standards initially in terms of what standards are unacceptable to you. Your standards may be influenced by role models whom you have identified as being particularly skilled in a certain area of practice. It may be helpful to note down these particular qualities to which you aspire. However, it is also useful to note that some practitioners define 'excellence' as being consistently good.[9] Indeed you may recognise that this is much harder to achieve (and demonstrate) than sporadic bursts of excellence.

This consistency is a critical factor in considering competence and performance too (*see* page 15). The documents that you collect in your evidence cycles must reflect consistency over time and in different circumstances, for example with various types of patients or your practice at different times of day. This will show that you have not only performed well on one occasion or for one type of baseline assessment, but also sustained your performance over time and under different conditions.

Stage 2: Set the standards for your outcomes – for being competent and providing a good service

Outcomes might include:

- the way that learning is applied
- a learnt skill
- a protocol
- a strategy that is implemented
- meeting recommended standards.

The level at which you should be performing depends on your particular field of expertise. Generalist nurses are good at seeing the wider picture, while specialists tend to be expert in a narrow area, so that the level of competence expected for a clinical area will vary depending on the nurse's role and responsibilities. You would not, for example, expect nurse specialists in women's health to be competent at managing patients with cardiac failure (although some of them may be), but you would expect practice nurses to be able to manage a wide variety of conditions, but with limited expertise in certain areas. You would expect both the specialist nurse and the generalist nurse to recognise their 'scope of professional practice'[10] and to refer to someone with more expertise when necessary.

Other standards include using resources effectively and the record keeping that is an essential tool in clinical care. As a health professional, you need to be accessible and available so that you can provide your services, and make suitable arrangements for handing over care to others. You could incorporate into your standards or outcomes those components specified by universities at a national level as part of their Masters Frameworks for their postgraduate awards. The Masters Frameworks consist of eight components that shape the individual postgraduate award programme outcomes and the learning outcomes of the individual modules for the postgraduate awards. The eight components are shown in Box 1.3. You could set out your CPD work in the portfolio you are assembling for re-registration and your annual appraisals in this format. This would help you to document your professional development to date in a form that can be readily 'accredited for prior experiential learning' (APEL) by universities (contact your local universities if you want more information about this process). You might then be given credits for learning against an intended postgraduate award. It would save you from duplicating work as well as speeding your progress through the award.

Box 1.3:   The eight components of the Masters Frameworks for postgraduate awards

1 Analysis
2 Problem solving
3 Knowledge and understanding
4 Reflection
5 Communication

> 6 Learning
> 7 Application
> 8 Enquiry

If you have information or data about your work showing that it was substandard or that you were not competent, you might choose to exclude that from your portfolio. However, you will be able to show that you have learnt more by reviewing mistakes or negative episodes. It is better to include everything of relevance, then go on to demonstrate how you addressed the gaps in your performance and made sustained improvements. You will need to protect the confidentiality of patients and colleagues as necessary when you collect data. The NMC will be seeing the contents of your re-registration portfolio if your submission is one of those sampled. You will probably also submit or share the documentation for job interviews and for your appraisal and maybe use it for reviews within clinical supervision sessions.

Stage 3: Identify your learning and service needs in your work or trust and rank them in order of priority[3]

The type and depth of documentation you need to gather will encompass:

* the context in which you work
* your knowledge and skills in relation to any particular role or responsibility of your current post.

The extent of expertise you should possess will depend on your level of responsibility for a particular function or task. You may be personally responsible for that function or task, or you may contribute or delegate responsibility for it. Your learning needs should take into account your aspirations for the future too – personal or career development for you, or improvements in the way you deliver care in your practice. Look at Chapter 2 for more ideas on how you will identify your learning or service development needs.

Group and summarise your service development needs from the exercises you have carried out. Grade them according to the priority you set. You may put one at a higher priority because it fits in with service development needs established in the business plan of the trust or practice, or put another lower because it does not fit in with other activities that your organisation has in their current development plan for the next 12 months. If you have identified a service development need by various methods of assessment, or with several different patient groups or clinical conditions, then it will have a higher priority than something only identified once. Notify the service development needs you have identified to those responsible for agreeing and implementing the development plans of the trust and/or practice.

Look back at your aspirations and standards set out in Stages 1 and 2. Match your learning or service development needs with one or more of these standards, or others that you have set yourself.

Stage 4: Make and carry out a learning and action plan with a timetable for your personal and service development

If you have not identified any learning needs for yourself or the service as a whole, you should omit Stage 4 and tidy up the presentation of your evidence for inclusion in your portfolio as at the end of Stage 5.

Think about whether:

- you have defined your learning objectives – what you need to learn to be able to attain the standards and outcomes you have described in Stage 2
- you can justify spending time and effort on the topics you prioritised in Stage 3. Is the topic important enough to your work, the NHS as a whole or patient safety? Does the clinical or non-clinical event occur sufficiently often to warrant the time spent?
- the time and resources for learning about that topic or making the associated changes to service delivery are available. Check that you are not trying to do too much too quickly, or you will become discouraged
- learning about that topic will make a difference to the care you or others can provide for patients
- and how one topic fits in with other topics you have identified to learn more about. Have you achieved a good balance across your areas of work or between your personal aspirations and the basic requirements of the service?

Decide on what method of learning is most appropriate for your task or role or the standards you are expecting to attain or sustain. You may have already identified your preferred learning style – but read up on this elsewhere if you are unsure.

Describe how you will carry out your learning tasks and what you will do by a specified time. State how your learning will be applied and how and when it will be evaluated. Build in some staging posts so that you do not suddenly get to the end of 12 months and discover that you have only done half of your plan.

Your action plan should also include your role in remedying any gaps in service delivery that you identified in Stage 3 that are within the remit of your responsibility.

Stage 5: Document your learning, competence, performance and standards of service delivery

You might choose to document that you have attained your defined outcomes by repeating the learning needs assessment that you started with. You could record your increased confidence and competence in dealing with situations that you previously avoided or performed inadequately.

You might incorporate your assessment of what has been gained in a study of another area that overlaps.

Preparing your portfolio

Use your portfolio of evidence of what you have learnt and your standards of practice to:

- identify significant experiences to serve as important sources of learning
- reflect on the learning that arose from those experiences
- demonstrate learning in practice
- analyse and identify further learning needs and ways in which these needs can be met.

Your documentation might include all sorts of things, not just formal audits – although they make a good start. It might include reports of educational activities attended, statements of your roles and responsibilities, copies of publications you have read and critically appraised, and reports of your work. You could incorporate observations by others, evaluations of you observing other colleagues and how their practice differs from yours, descriptions of self-improvements, a video of typical activity, materials that demonstrate your skills to others, products of your input or learning – a new protocol for example. Box 1.4 gives a list of material you might include in your portfolio.

Box 1.4:   Possible contents of a portfolio

- Workload logs
- Case descriptions
- Videos
- Audiotapes
- Patient satisfaction surveys
- Research surveys
- Report of change or innovation
- Commentaries on published literature or books
- Records of critical incidents and learning points
- Notes from formal teaching sessions with reference to clinical work or other evidence

---

When you are preparing to submit your portfolio for a discussion with your manager (for example, at an appraisal) or for an assessment (for example, for a university post-registration award), write a self-assessment of your previous action plan. You might integrate your self-assessment into your PDP to show what you have achieved and what gaps you have still to address. Decide where you are now and where you want to be in one, three or five years' time.

Make sure all references are included and the documentation in your portfolio is as accurate and complete as possible. Organise how you have shown your learning steps and your standards of practice so that it is indexed and cross-referenced to the relevant sections of the paperwork. Discuss the contents of your portfolio with a colleague or a mentor to gain other people's perspectives of your work and look for blind spots.

Reflective writing within the portfolio

Reflective writing has been endorsed by the NMC as an excellent way of analysing practice and learning from your everyday experiences.[2] Reflective writing can also be useful to analyse what you have learnt from attending formal learning sessions and considering how any newly acquired knowledge may be applied to practice. In order to provide a comprehensive structure to reflective writing it is recommended that a model of reflection is adopted. This will help you to learn from your experience in a more logical and holistic manner. There are numerous models of reflection and it is best to choose a model which appears straightforward to you and seems to fit with your own style of thinking.[11–13]

Reflective writing introduces a personal element into your portfolio. It enables anyone reading the portfolio to gain insight into your practice. It is useful in creating a picture, which gives access to the artistry of nursing, and may demonstrate the therapeutic use of self in patient interactions.

Include evidence of your competence as a practitioner with a special interest

You may have a particular expertise or special interest in a clinical field or non-clinical area such as management, teaching or research. It may be that you have a lead role or responsibility in your practice for chronic disease management of clinical conditions such as diabetes, asthma, mental health or coronary heart disease or as a community matron with responsibility for case management of patients with long-term conditions and high-intensity needs.[14] You may be employed by a PCO or hospital trust to:

- lead in the development of services
- deliver a procedure-based service
- deliver an opinion-based service.

The role of practitioner with special interest (PwSI) is being promoted as a role to help to bridge the gap between hospital and the community.[14] Realising the potential of nurses and allied health professionals working in specialist roles will facilitate the redesign of primary care services. It may be particularly important for you, as a specialist, to be able to demonstrate your clinical expertise if you are seeking to gain a position as a PwSI. There is little consistency in the extent of training or qualifications at present within or across the various PwSI specialty areas.[14] Whatever your role, responsibility or expertise, your portfolio should include examples of evidence that show that you are competent, and that you have a consistently good performance in your specialty area. You may have parallel appraisals that you can include from your employer – for example, the university if you have a research or teaching post, or a hospital consultant if he or she supervises you in the clinical specialty.

When you gather evidence of your performance at work, try to document as many aspects of your work at one time as you can. When you are identifying what you need to learn, or gaps in service delivery, make sure that you involve patients and show how you interact with the team. This gives you evidence about 'relationships with patients' and 'working with colleagues' as well as the clinical area that you are focusing on or auditing.

References

1   Nursing and Midwifery Council (2002) *Code of Professional Conduct.* Nursing and Midwifery Council, London.

2   Nursing and Midwifery Council (2001) *The PREP Handbook.* Nursing and Midwifery Council, London.

3   Wakley G, Chambers R and Field S (2000) *Continuing Professional Development in Primary Care.* Radcliffe Medical Press, Oxford.

4   Department of Health (2004) *The NHS Knowledge and Skills Framework (NHS KSF) and the Development Review Process.* Department of Health, London.

5   Brown R (1995) *Portfolio Development and Profiling for Nurses* (2e). Quay Publishing, Wiltshire.

6   English National Board for Nursing, Midwifery and Health Visiting (1997) *Standards for Approval of Higher Education Institutions and Programmes.* English National Board for Nursing, Midwifery and Health Visiting, London.

7   Quinn F (2000) *Principles and Practice of Nurse Education* (4e). Stanley Thornes Ltd, London.

8   Nursing and Midwifery Council (2002) *Supporting Nurses and Midwives through Lifelong Learning.* Nursing and Midwifery Council, London.

9   Royal College of General Practitioners/General Practitioners Committee (2002) *Good Medical Practice for General Practitioners.* Royal College of General Practitioners, London.

10 Nursing and Midwifery Council (1992) *Scope of Professional Practice.* Nursing and Midwifery Council, London.

11 Gibbs G (1998) *Learning by Doing: a guide to teaching and learning methods.* Further Education Unit, Oxford Polytechnic, London.

12 Johns C (1996) Using a reflective model of nursing and guided reflection. *Nursing Standard.* **11(2)**: 34–8.

13 Schon D (1983) *The Reflective Practitioner: how professionals think in action.* Basic Books, New York.

14 Department of Health (2003) *Practitioners with Special Interests in Primary Care: implementing a scheme for nurses with special interests in primary care.* Department of Health, London. www.dh.gov.uk/assetRoot/04/06/92/07/04069207.pdf (accessed 25 April 2005)

2

Practical ways to identify your learning and service needs as part of your portfolio

Setting standards to show that you are competent

The Nursing and Midwifery Council (NMC) stresses the importance of lifelong learning. The Council recognises that healthcare is an area of constant change which necessitates a dynamic approach to learning. In order to develop and maintain your competence you are required to 'demonstrate responsibility for your own learning through the development of a portfolio ... and to be able to recognise when further learning and development may be required'.[1]

You could make a good start by describing your current roles and responsibilities. This will help you to define what your competence should be now, or what competence you are hoping to attain (for instance as a specialist nurse). Once you have your definition, you can recognise whether you have, or lack in some part, the necessary competence. If there are no accepted descriptions of competence in the area you are focusing on, then you will have to start from scratch. You might compile your description using items from national guidelines such as in the National Service Frameworks or health strategies or Agenda for Change.[2] The Department of Health has produced ideas relating to the role of nurses with special interests that you may find useful to adopt.[3]

Your definition of competence is likely to relate to your ability to undertake a task or role to a required standard. However, you will need to describe the standards expected in the range of tasks and roles you undertake, and reference the source of standard setting. If professionals, or their organisations, are the only people involved in setting those standards, consider whether you should amend or extend the standards, tasks or roles by considering other perspectives, such as those of patients or your employing trust or practice.

There is a difference between being competent, and performing in a consistently competent manner. You need to be motivated to perform consistently well and enabled to do so with efficient systems and sufficient resources. You will require sufficient numbers of other competent healthcare professionals and available infrastructure such as diagnostic and treatment resources. It is partially your responsibility to alert managers to the resources needed to undertake your role effectively.

Choose methods in Stage 3 (*see* Chapter 1) to demonstrate your standards of performance and identify any learning needs that span different topic areas, to reduce duplication and maximise the usefulness of your learning. Collecting evidence of more than one aspect of your competence or performance cuts down the overall amount of work underpinning your PDP or included in your appraisal portfolio.

Use several methods to identify your learning needs and/or gaps in your service development or delivery, so that you validate the findings of one method by another. No one method will give you reliable information about the gaps in your knowledge, skills or attitudes or everyday service. Does what you think about your performance match with what others in the team or patients think of how you practise in your everyday work? It is particularly difficult to determine what it is you 'don't know you don't know' by yourself, yet it is vital that you identify and rectify those gaps. Other people may be able to tell you what you need to learn quite readily. Colleagues from different disciplines could usefully comment on any shortfalls in how your work interfaces with theirs.

Patients or people who don't use your services could tell you whether the way you work or provide services is off-putting or inappropriate. There may be data about your performance or your approach that could point out those gaps in your knowledge or skills of which you were previously unaware.

Determine what it is that you 'don't know you don't know' by:

- asking patients, users and non-users of your service
- comparing your performance against best practice or that of peers
- comparing your performance against objectives in business plans or national directives
- asking colleagues from different disciplines about shortfalls in how your work interfaces with theirs.

Identify your learning needs – how you can find out if you need to be better at doing your job

You may decide to use a few selected methods to gather baseline evidence of your performance, focused on your specific area of expertise. Once you have identified your learning needs you will be able to create a flexible way to progress that takes account of your needs and circumstances. In order to establish your current position with a degree of objectivity you might use several of the methods described in this chapter such as:

- constructive feedback from peers or patients
- 360° feedback

- self-assessment, or review by others, using a rating scale to assess your skills and attitudes
- comparison with local or national protocols and guidelines for checking how well procedures are followed
- evaluative audit
- significant event audit
- eliciting patient views through methods such as satisfaction surveys
- a SWOT (strengths, weaknesses, opportunities and threats) or SCOT (strengths, challenges, opportunities and threats) analysis
- reading and reflecting
- educational review.

Several of these methods will also be useful for identifying any service development needs – you can look at the gaps identified from both the personal and service perspectives at the same time using the same method.

Seek feedback

Find colleagues who will give you constructive feedback about your performance and practice. Don't be afraid to ask for comments on your style or work – just think how upsetting it would be if you were consistently doing something that irritated colleagues, but continued because nobody bothered to tell you the effect it was having. The golden rule for giving constructive feedback is to give positive praise of things that have been well done first. Sometimes colleagues launch straight in to criticise faults when asked for their views. The Pendleton model of the giving of feedback is widely used in the health setting (*see* Box 2.1):[4]

Box 2.1: The Pendleton model of giving feedback

1 The 'learner' goes first and performs the activity.
2 The 'teacher' questions or clarifies any facts.
3 The 'learner' says what they thought was done well.
4 The 'teacher' says what they thought was done well.
5 The 'learner' says what could be improved upon.
6 The 'teacher' says what could be improved upon.
7 Both discuss ideas for improvements in a helpful and constructive manner.

360° feedback

This collects together perceptions from a number of different participants as shown in Figure 2.1.

The wider the spread of people giving feedback, the more rounded the picture. Each individual gives a feedback questionnaire to at least three people in each of the groups above. An independent person then collects and collates the questionnaires and discusses the results with the individual. Computerised versions are available from commercial companies.[5] The main disadvantage of this method is that it can sometimes

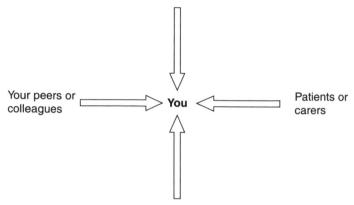

Figure 2.1:   360° feedback.

be spoilt by malicious comments against which individuals cannot readily defend themselves.

Self-assess or gain another person's perspective on your standard of practice or service delivery

You might describe any aspect of your practice as statements (A to G as in Box 2.2) about your competence or performance for you to self-assess or others to give you feedback or comments by marking the extent to which they agree on the linear scales opposite. Objective feedback from external assessment is usually more reliable than your own self-assessment when you may have blind spots about your own performance. As you become more confident in this method of reviewing your competence, you might emphasise how consistent you are in your application of good practice – so in the statements below we have sometimes included 'consistently', 'always' or 'usually'. You can set your own challenges. If you have a mentor or a 'buddy' in the practice with whom you learn, you might discuss and reflect on the completed marking grids with him or her.

Box 2.2:   Marking grid: circle the number which represents your views or feelings about each statement – complete the grid on more than one occasion and compare results over time

A   I consistently treat patients politely and with consideration.

STRONGLY AGREE   to   STRONGLY DISAGREE

1----------------2----------------3----------------4----------------5----------------6

B   I am aware of how my personal beliefs could affect the care offered to the patient, and take care not to impose my own beliefs and values.

STRONGLY AGREE   to   STRONGLY DISAGREE

1----------------2----------------3----------------4----------------5----------------6

C   I always treat all patients equally and ensure that some groups are not favoured at the expense of others.

STRONGLY AGREE   to   STRONGLY DISAGREE

1----------------2----------------3----------------4----------------5----------------6

D   I try to maintain a relationship with the patient or family when a mistake has occurred.

STRONGLY AGREE   to   STRONGLY DISAGREE

1----------------2----------------3----------------4----------------5----------------6

E   I always obtain informed consent to treatment.

STRONGLY AGREE   to   STRONGLY DISAGREE

1----------------2----------------3----------------4----------------5----------------6

F   I usually involve patients in decisions about their care.

STRONGLY AGREE   to   STRONGLY DISAGREE

1----------------2----------------3----------------4----------------5----------------6

G   I always respect the right of patients to refuse treatments or tests.

STRONGLY AGREE   to   STRONGLY DISAGREE

1----------------2----------------3----------------4----------------5----------------6

Compare your performance against protocols or guidelines

Are you familiar with all the protocols or guidelines that are used by someone, somewhere in your team? You might determine your learning needs and those of other team members by piling all the protocols or guidelines that exist in your team in a big heap and rationalising them so that you have a common set used by all. Working as a team you can compare your own knowledge and usual practice with others and with protocols or guidelines recommended by the National Institute for Clinical Excellence (NICE)[6] or National Service Frameworks or the Scottish Intercollegiate Guidelines Network (SIGN).[7]

Alternatively, you might compare your own practice against a protocol or guideline that is generally accepted at a national or local level. You could audit the standard of your practice to find out how often you adhere to such a protocol or guideline, and if you can justify why you deviate from the recommendations.

Audit

Audit is:

> the method used by health professionals to assess, evaluate, and improve the care of patients in a systematic way, to enhance their health and quality of life.[8]

The five steps of the audit cycle are shown in Box 2.3.

Box 2.3:   The five steps of the audit cycle

1   Describe the criteria and standards you are trying to achieve.
2   Measure your current performance of how well you are providing care or services in an objective way.
3   Compare your performance against criteria and standards.
4   Identify the need for change – to performance, adjustment of criteria or standards, resources, available data.
5   Make any required changes as necessary and re-audit later.

Performance or practice is often broken down for the purposes of audit into the three aspects of structure, process and outcome. Structural audits might concern resources such as equipment, premises, skills, people, etc. Process audits focus on what is done to the patient: for instance, clinical protocols and guidelines. Audits of outcomes consider the impact of care or services on the patient and might include patient satisfaction, health gains and effectiveness of care or services. You might look at aspects of quality of the structure, process and outcome of the delivery of any clinical field – focusing on access, equity of care between different groups in the population, efficiency, economy, effectiveness for individual patients, etc.[8]

Set standards for your performance, find out how you are doing, search to find out best practice, make the changes and then re-audit the care given to patients in the future with the same problem. Some variations on audit include:

- *case note analysis*. This gives an insight into your current practice. It might be a retrospective review of a random selection of notes, or a prospective survey of consecutive patients with the same condition as they present to see you
- *peer review*. Compare an area of practice with other individual professionals or managers; or compare practice teams as a whole. An independent body might compare all practices in one area e.g. within a PCO so that like is compared with

like. Feedback may be arranged to protect participants' identities so that only the individual person or practice knows their own identity, the rest being anonymised, for example by giving each practice a number. Where there is mutual trust and an open learning culture, peer review does not need to be anonymised and everyone can learn together about making improvements in practice

- *criteria-based audit*. This compares clinical practice with specific standards, guidelines or protocols. Re-audit of changes should demonstrate improvements in the quality of patient care
- *external audit*. Prescribing advisers or managers in PCOs can supply information about indicators of performance for audit. Visits from external bodies such as the Healthcare Commission expose the PCO or hospital trust in England and Wales to external audit
- *tracer criteria*. Assessing the quality of care of a 'tracer' condition may be used to represent the quality of care of other similar conditions or more complex problems. Tracer criteria should be easily defined and measured. For instance, if you were to audit the extent to which you reviewed the treatment of asthma, you might focus on a drug such as beclometasone and generalise from your audit results to your likely performance with other medications.

Significant event audit

Think of an incident where a patient or you experienced an adverse event. This might be an unexpected death, an unplanned pregnancy, an avoidable side-effect from prescribed medication, a violent attack on a member of staff, or an angry outburst in public by you or a work colleague. You can review the case and reflect on the sequence of events that led to that critical event occurring. It is likely that there were a multitude of factors leading up to that significant event. You should take the case to a multi-disciplinary meeting to reflect and analyse what were the triggers, causes and consequences of the event. Complete the significant event audit cycle by planning what individuals or the healthcare team as a whole might do to avoid a similar event happening in future. This might include undertaking further learning and/or making appropriate changes to your systems.

The steps of a significant event audit are shown in Box 2.4.

Box 2.4:　Steps of a significant event audit

- *Step 1*: Describe who was involved, what time of day, what the task/activity was, the context and any other relevant information.
- *Step 2*: Reflect on the effects of the event on the participants and the professionals involved.
- *Step 3*: Discuss the reasons for the event or situation arising with other colleagues, review case notes or other records.
- *Step 4*: Decide how you or others might have behaved differently. Describe your options for how the procedures at work might be changed to minimise or eliminate the chances of the event recurring.

- *Step 5*: Plan changes that are needed, how they will be implemented, who will be responsible for what and when, what further training or resources are required. Then carry out the changes.
- *Step 6*: Re-audit later to see whether changes to procedures or new knowledge and skills are having the desired effects. Give feedback to the practice team.

An assessment by an external body

This is a traditional way of showing that you are competent by taking and passing an examination. It is a good way of testing recalled knowledge in a written or oral examination, or establishing how you behave in a clinical situation on the day of a practical examination, but not much good for measuring anything else. A summative examination (i.e. done at the end of a course of study) gives a measure of your learning up to that date.

You might undertake an objective test of your knowledge and skills. Examples are a computer-based test in the form of multiple choice questions and patient management problems as in the nurse prescribing website.[9] It may be worth considering subscribing to websites that provide multiple choice questionnaires that you can complete on paper (e.g. Guidelines in Practice[10]) and record this in your portfolio.

Elicit the views of patients

In striving to establish consistently good relationships with patients you may assess patients' satisfaction with:

- you
- your practice
- the local hospital's way of working
- other services available in your locality.

Avoid surveys where questions are relatively superficial or biased. A more specific enquiry should uncover particular elements of patients' dissatisfaction, which will be more useful if you are trying to identify your learning needs. Use a well-validated patient questionnaire instead of risking producing your own version with ambiguities and flaws such as the General Practice Assessment Questionnaire (GPAQ).[11] Many health professionals have used these patient survey methods, providing a bank of data against which to compare your performance.

Other sources of feedback from patients might be obtained through suggestion boxes for patients to contribute comments, or ask the team to record all patients' suggestions and complaints, however trivial, looking for patterns in the comments received.

There will be learning to be had from every complaint – even if the complaint does not have any substance, there should be something to learn about the shortfall in communication between you and the complainant.

The evolution of the 'expert patient programme' should mean that there is a pool of well informed patients with chronic conditions who can contribute their insights into what you (or the service) need to learn from a patient's perspective.[12]

Strengths, weaknesses (or challenges), opportunities and threats (SWOT or SCOT) analysis

You can undertake a SWOT (or SCOT) analysis of your own performance or that of your nursing team or healthcare organisation, working it out on your own, or with a workmate or mentor, or with a group of colleagues. Brainstorm the strengths, weaknesses (or challenges), opportunities and threats of your role or circumstances.

Strengths and weaknesses (or challenges) of your roles might relate to your clinical knowledge or skills, experience, expertise, decision making, communication skills, inter-professional relationships, political skills, timekeeping, organisational skills, teaching skills, or research skills. Strengths and weaknesses (or challenges) of the practice organisation might relate to most of these aspects as well as the way resources are allocated, overall efficiency and the degree to which the practice is patient centred.

Opportunities might relate to your unexploited experience or potential strengths, expected changes in the NHS, or resources for which you might bid. For example, you might train for and set up a special interest post.

Threats will include factors and circumstances that prevent you from achieving your aims for personal, professional and practice development or service improvements. They might be to do with your health, turnover in the team, or time-limited investment by your employing organisation.

List the important factors in your SWOT (or SCOT) analysis in order of priority through discussion with colleagues and independent people from outside your practice. Draw up goals and a timed action plan for you or the practice team to follow.

Informal conversations – in the corridor, over coffee

You learn such a lot when chatting with colleagues at coffee time or over a meal and can become aware of your learning or service development needs at these times. This is when you realise that other people are doing things differently from you and if they seem to be doing it better and achieving more, you can challenge yourself to decide if this matter could be one of your blind spots. Note down your thoughts before you forget them so that you can reflect on them later.

Online discussion groups may provide another source of informal exchanges with colleagues. If you find this difficult to start with, you might 'lurk', viewing the comments and views of other people until you feel confident enough to contribute. Record any observations that you find useful and reflect on how they might inform your own practice.

Observe your work environment and role

Observation could be informal and opportunistic, or more systematic working through a structured checklist. One method of self-assessment might be to audiotape yourself at work dealing with patients (after obtaining patients' informed consent). Listen to the tape afterwards to appraise your communication and consultation skills – on your own or with a friend or colleague. If you have access to video equipment, you might use this instead. You would need to discuss this in advance with your manager and comply with any policies on consent and confidentiality.

Look at the equipment that you use within your daily work. Do you know how to operate it properly? Assess yourself undertaking practical procedures or ask someone to watch you operating the equipment or undertaking a practical procedure, and give you feedback about your performance.

Analyse the various roles and responsibilities of your current posts. Compare your level of expertise against national standards such as in the Knowledge and Skills Framework (KSF) or job evaluation framework as part of the Agenda for Change initiative.[13,14] Determine whether you can meet the requirements, or, if not, what deficiencies need to be made good.

You might combine one of the methods of identifying your learning needs already described such as an audit or SWOT analysis and apply it to 'observing your work environment or role', describing your relationship with other members of the multidisciplinary team for example, or reviewing how their roles and responsibilities interface with yours.

Read and reflect

When reading articles in respected journals, reflect on what the key messages mean for you in your situation. Note down topics about which you know little but that are relevant to your work and calculate if you have further learning needs not met by the article you are reading. If the article is relevant to your work, record what changes you will make and how you will make the changes. Record how you will impart your new knowledge to others in your workplace.

Educational review

You might find a buddy or work colleague, clinical tutor, or a clinical tutor or clinical supervisor with whom you can have an informal or formal discussion about your performance, job situation and learning needs. You might draw up a learning contract as a result with a timed plan of action.

Identify your service needs – how you can find out if there are gaps in services or how you deliver care

Now focus your attention on the needs of your practice or of your service organisation. The standards of service delivery should be those that allow you to practise as a competent clinician. You may be competent but be unable to perform or practise to a competent level if the resources available to you are inadequate, or other colleagues have insufficient knowledge or skills to support you. You cannot be expected to take responsibility for ensuring that resources you need to be able to practise in a competent manner are available. However, as a professional you should play a significant role in collecting evidence to make a case for the need for essential resources to your manager.

Some of the methods you might use are described below and include:

- involving patients and the public in giving you feedback about the quality and quantity of your services
- monitoring access to and availability of care
- undertaking a force-field analysis
- assessing risk
- evaluating the standards of care or services you provide
- comparing the systems in your practice with those required by legislation
- considering your patient population's health needs
- reviewing teamwork
- assessing the quality of your services
- reflecting on whether you are providing cost-effective care and services.

Involve patients and the public in giving you feedback about the quality and quantity of your services

Patient and public involvement may occur at three levels:

1 for individual patients about their own care
2 for patients and the public about the range and quality of health services on offer
3 in planning and organising health service developments.

The phrase 'patient and public involvement' is used here to mean individual involvement as a user, patient or carer, or public involvement that includes the processes of consultation and participation.[15]

If a patient involvement or public consultation exercise is to be meaningful, it has to involve people who represent the section of the population that the exercise is about. You will have to set up systems to actively seek out and involve people from minority groups or those with sensory impairments such as blind and deaf people.

Before you start:

- define the purpose
- be realistic about the magnitude of the planned exercise

- select an appropriate method or several methods depending on the target population and your resources
- obtain the commitment of everyone who will be affected by the exercise
- frame the method in accordance with your perspective
- write the protocol.

You might hold focus groups, or set up a patient panel, or invite feedback and help from a patient participation group. You could interview patients selected either at random from the patient population or for their experience of a particular condition or circumstance.

Monitor access to and availability of healthcare

Access and availability

You could look at waiting times to see a health professional by using:

- computerised appointment lists or paper and pen to record the time of arrival, the time of the appointment, the time seen
- the next available appointments that can easily be monitored by computer, or more painfully by manual searches of the appointment books.

Compare the results at intervals (a spreadsheet is a good way to do this). Do you or your staff have learning needs in relation to the use of technology, or new ways of redesigning the service you offer?

Referrals to other agencies and hospitals

You might audit and re-audit the time taken from the date the patient is seen to:

- the referral being sent (do you need more secretarial time?)
- the date the patient is seen by the other agency (could the patient be seen elsewhere quicker or do you need to liaise with other agencies over referrals?)
- the date the patient's needs have been met by investigation, diagnosis, treatment, provision of aid or support, etc (can you influence how quickly these are completed?).

Identify any learning needs here. For instance, new methods of teamwork with a different mix of skills between nurses, doctors and allied health professionals could provide extra services for your patients.

Draw up a force-field analysis

This tool will help you to identify and focus down on the positive and negative forces in your work and to gain an overview of the weighting of these factors. Draw a horizontal or vertical line in the middle of a sheet of paper. Label one side 'positive' and the other side 'negative'. Draw bars to represent individual positive drivers that motivate you on one side of the line, and factors that are demotivating on the other negative side of the line. The thickness and length of the bars should represent the extent of the influence;

that is, a short, narrow bar will indicate that the positive or negative factor has a minor influence and a long, wide bar a major effect. *See* Box 2.5 for an example.

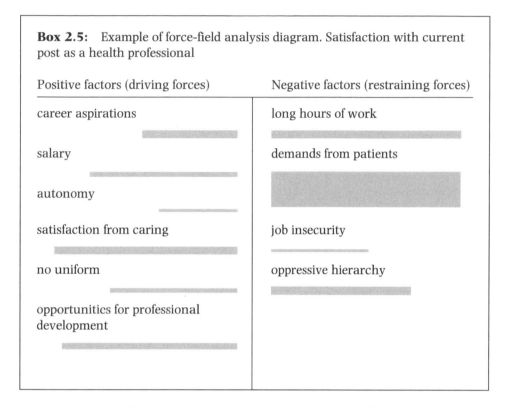

Box 2.5:   Example of force-field analysis diagram. Satisfaction with current post as a health professional

Positive factors (driving forces)	Negative factors (restraining forces)
career aspirations	long hours of work
salary	demands from patients
autonomy	
satisfaction from caring	job insecurity
no uniform	oppressive hierarchy
opportunities for professional development	

Take an overview of the resulting force-field diagram and consider if you are content with things as they are, or can think of ways to boost the positive side and minimise the negative factors. You can do this part of the exercise on your own, with a peer or a small group in the practice, or with a mentor or someone from outside the workplace. The exercise should help you to realise the extent to which a known influence in your life, or in the practice as a whole, is a positive or negative factor. Make a personal or organisational action plan to create the situations and opportunities to boost the positive factors in your life and minimise the bars on the negative side.

Assess risk

Risk assessment might entail evaluating the risks to the health or wellbeing or competence of yourself, staff and/or patients in your practice or workplace, and deciding on the action needed to minimise or eliminate those risks.[16] Risk assessment is part of the clinical governance framework of your organisation, which should have a standard process for reporting and reviewing adverse incidents, which may alert you to hazards through a root cause analysis where you aim to identify the fundamental cause(s) of the adverse event.

- *A hazard*: something with the potential to cause harm.
- *A risk*: the likelihood of that potential to cause harm being realised.

There are five steps to risk assessment:

1. look for and list the hazards
2. decide who might be harmed and how
3. evaluate the risks arising from the hazards and decide whether existing precautions are adequate or more should be done
4. record the findings
5. review your assessment from time to time and revise it if necessary.

You do not want to spend a lot of time and effort identifying risks or making changes if they do not matter much. When you have identified a risk, consider:

- is the risk large?
- does it happen often?
- is it a significant risk?

Risks may be prevented, avoided, minimised or managed where they cannot be eliminated. You, your colleagues and your staff may need to learn how to do this.

Record significant events where someone has experienced an adverse event or had a near miss – as part of you identifying your service development needs on an ongoing basis. Most significant incidents do not have one cause. Usually there are faults in the system, which are compounded by someone or several people being careless, tired, overworked or ill-informed. Cultivate an atmosphere of openness and discussion without blame so that you can all learn from the significant event. If people think they will be blamed they will hide the incident and no one will be able to prevent it happening again. Look for *all* the causes and try to remedy as many as possible to prevent the situation from arising in the future.

Evaluate the standards of services or care you provide

Keep your evaluation as simple as possible. Avoid wasting resources on unnecessarily bureaucratic evaluation. Design the evaluation so that you:

- specify the event (such as a service) to be evaluated – define broad issues, set priorities against strategic goals, time and resources, seek agreement on the nature and scope of the task
- describe the expected impact of the programme or activity and who will be affected
- define the criteria of success – these might relate to structure, process or outcome
- identify the information required to demonstrate the achievements of the programme or activity. The record might include: observing behaviour; data from existing records; prospective recording by the subjects of the programme or by the recipients and staff of the activity
- determine the time frame for the evaluation

- specify who collects the data for all stages in the delivery of the programme or activity, and the respective deadlines
- review and refine the objectives of the programme or activity and check that they are appropriate for the outcomes and impact you expect.

What to evaluate?

You could:

- adopt any, or all, of the six aspects of the health service's performance assessment framework: health improvement, fair access, effective delivery, efficiency, patient/ carer experience, health outcomes
- agree milestones and goals at stages in your programme or adopt others such as relate to the National Service Frameworks
- evaluate the extent to which you achieve the outcome(s) starting with an objective. Alternatively, you might evaluate how conducive is the context of the programme, or activity, to achieving the anticipated outcomes
- undertake regular audits of aspects of the structure, process and outcome of a service or project to see if you have achieved what you expected when you established the criteria and standards of the audit programme
- evaluate the various components of a new system or programme: the activities, personnel involved, provision of services, organisational structure, precise goals and interventions.

Computer search

The extent to which you can evaluate the practice of the healthcare team will depend on the quality of your records and the extent to which you use a computer to record healthcare information. In a general practice setting, for example, you could undertake a computerised search to identify those patients on treatment for diabetes who have attended a diabetic clinic within the practice over the past six months. In a hospital setting, you could compare the duration of stay for patients undergoing particular surgery and analyse the reasons for variance. Make appropriate changes to your systems depending on what the computer search reveals. Put your plan into action and monitor with repeat searches at regular intervals.

Look at your learning or service development needs by analysing data from your records to:

- look at trends and patterns of illness
- devise and use clinical guidelines and decision support systems as part of evidence-based practice
- audit what you are doing
- provide the information on which to base decisions on commissioning and management
- support epidemiology, research and teaching activities.

Compare the systems in your workplace with those required by legislation

Legislation changes quite frequently. If you are employed within a large organisation such as an acute hospital you can rely on managers to cascade information relating to legislative requirements down to you. In smaller organisations, such as general practice settings, you may need to raise awareness of legislative requirements. You could start by comparing the systems in your practice or workplace with those required by the Disability Discrimination Act (1995) and health and safety legislation.

Consider your patients' health needs

Create a detailed profile of the local community that you serve. Ask your PCO or public health lead for information about practice populations and comparative information about the general population living in the district – morbidity and mortality statistics, referral patterns, age/sex mix, ethnicity, and population trends. You could also liaise with the wider community nursing service to investigate what information they hold relating to the health of the community.

Include information about the wider determinants of health such as housing, numbers of the population in, and types of, employment, geographical location, the environment, crime and safety, educational attainment and socio-economic data. Make a note of any particular health problems such as higher than average teenage pregnancy rates or drug misuse. If you work in a general practice setting you could focus on the current state of health inequalities within your practice population or between your practice population and the district as a whole. It may be that circumstances change, which in turn alters the proportion of minority groups in a local area such as if new continuing care homes open up, or there is an influx of homeless people or asylum seekers into the locality.

Review teamwork

You can measure how effective the team is[17] – evaluate whether the team has:

- clear goals and objectives
- accountability and authority
- individual roles for members
- shared tasks
- regular internal formal and informal communication
- full participation by members
- confrontation of conflict
- feedback to individuals
- feedback about team performance
- outside recognition
- two-way external communication
- team rewards.

Assess the quality of your services

Quality may be subdivided into eight components: equity, access, acceptability and responsiveness, appropriateness, communication, continuity, effectiveness and efficiency.[18]

You might use the matrix in Box 2.6 as a way of ordering your approach to auditing a particular topic with the eight aspects of quality on the vertical axis and structure, process and outcome on the horizontal axis.[19] In this way you can generate up to 24 aspects of a particular topic. You might then focus on several aspects to look at the quality of patient care or services from various angles.

Box 2.6: Matrix for assessing the quality of a clinical service

You might look at the structure, process or outcome of communicating test results to patients for example.

	Structure	Process	Outcome
Equity			
Access			
Acceptability and responsiveness			
Appropriateness			
Communication	Hospital report	Feedback	Action taken
Continuity			
Effectiveness			
Efficiency			

Look for service development needs reflecting why patients receive a poor quality of service such as:

- inadequately trained staff or staff with poor levels of competence
- lack of confidentiality
- staff not being trained in the management of emergency situations
- doctors or nurses not being contactable in an emergency or being ineffective
- treatment being unavailable due to poor management of resources or services
- poor management of the arrangements for home visiting
- insufficient numbers of available staff for the workload
- qualifications of locums or deputising staff being unknown or inadequate for the posts they are filling
- arrangements for transfer of information from one team member to another being inadequate
- team members not acting on information received.

Many of these items will need action as a team, but for some of them, it may be your responsibility to ensure that adequate standards are met.

Reflect on whether you are providing cost-effective care and services

Cost-effectiveness is not synonymous with 'cheap'. A cost-effective intervention is one which gives a better or equivalent benefit from the intervention in question for lower or equivalent cost, or where the relative improvement in outcome is higher than the relative difference in cost. In other words being cost-effective means having the best outcomes for the least input. Using the term 'cost-effective' implies that you have considered potential alternatives.

An intervention must first be considered *clinically* effective to warrant investigation into its potential to be *cost*-effective. Evidence-based practice must incorporate clinical judgement. You have to interpret the evidence when it comes to applying it to individual patients, whether it is evidence about clinical effectiveness or cost-effectiveness. A new or alternative treatment or intervention should be compared directly with the previous best treatment or intervention.

An economic evaluation is a comparative analysis of two or more alternatives in terms of their costs and consequences. There are four different types as shown in Box 2.7.

Box 2.7:   The four types of economic evaluation

1   *Cost-effectiveness analysis* is used to compare the effectiveness of two interventions with the same treatment objectives.
2   *Cost minimisation* compares the costs of alternative treatments that have identical health outcomes.
3   *Cost–utility analysis* enables the effects of alternative interventions to be measured against a combination of life expectancy and quality of life; common outcome measures are quality adjusted life years (QALYs) or health-related quality of life (hrqol).
4   *Cost–benefit analysis* is a technique designed to determine the feasibility of a project, plan, management or treatment by quantifying its costs and benefits. It is often difficult to determine these accurately in relation to health.

While health valuation is unavoidable, it cannot be objective. You will probably have learning needs around what subjective method is best to use.[20]

Efficiency is sometimes confused with effectiveness. Being efficient means obtaining the most quality from the least expenditure, or the required level of quality for the least expenditure. To measure efficiency you need to make a judgement about the level of quality of the 'purchase' and be able to relate it to 'price'. 'Price' alone does not measure efficiency. Quality is the indicator used in combination with price to assess if something is more efficient. So, cost-effectiveness is a measure of efficiency and suggests that costs have been related to effectiveness.

Consider if you have service development needs. Discuss whether:

- the current skill mix in your team is appropriate
- more cost-effective alternative types of delivery of care are available
- sufficient staff training exists for those taking on new roles and responsibilities.

Set priorities: how you match what's needed with what's possible

You and your colleagues will have been able to make a wish list after following the previous Stages 3A and 3B undertaking a variety of needs assessments. Group and summarise your learning and service development needs from the exercises you have carried out. Grade them according to the priority you set. You may put one at a higher priority because it fits in with learning needs established from another section, or put another lower because it does not fit in with other activities that you will put into your learning plan for the next 12 months. If you have identified a learning need by several different methods of assessment then it will have a higher priority than something only identified once in your PDP. Collect information from all the team, the patients, users and carers to feed back before you make a decision on how to progress. Remember to take external influences into account such as the National Service Frameworks, NICE guidance, governmental priorities, priorities of your primary care organisation, the content of the Local Delivery Plan, etc.

Select those topics that are tied into organisational priorities, have clear aims and objectives and are achievable within your time and resource constraints. When ranking topics for learning or action in order of priority (Stage 4) consider whether:

- the project aims and objectives are clearly defined
- the topic is important:
    - for the population served (e.g. the size of the problem and/or its severity)
    - for the skills, knowledge or attitudes of the individual or team
- it is feasible
- it is affordable
- it will make enough difference
- it fits in with other priorities.

You will still have more ideas than can possibly be implemented. Remember the highest priority – the health service is for patients that use it or who will do so in the future.

References

1   Nursing and Midwifery Council (2002) *Supporting Nurses and Midwives through Lifelong Learning.* Nursing and Midwifery Council, London.

2   www.rcn.org.uk/agendaforchange (accessed 25 April 2005)

3   Department of Health (2003) *Practitioners with Special Interests.* Department of Health, London.

4   Pendleton D, Schofield T, Tate P *et al.* (2003) *The New Consultation: developing doctor–patient communication.* Oxford University Press, Oxford.

5   King J (2002) Career focus: 360° appraisal. *BMJ.* **324**: S195.

6   National Institute for Clinical Excellence (NICE) www.nice.org.uk (accessed 25 April 2005)

7   Scottish Intercollegiate Guidelines Network (SIGN) www.sign.ac.uk (accessed 25 April 2005)

8   Irvine D and Irvine S (eds) (1991) *Making Sense of Audit.* Radcliffe Medical Press, Oxford.

9   www.nurse-prescriber.co.uk/mcq.htm (accessed 25 April 2005)

10   www.eguidelines.co.uk (accessed 25 April 2005)

11   www.npcrdc.man.ac.uk (accessed 25 April 2005)

12   Department of Health (2003) EPP Update Newsletter. Department of Health, London. *See* Expert Patient Programme on www.expertpatients.nhs.uk

13   Department of Health (2004) *The NHS Knowledge and Skills Framework (NHS KSF) and the Development Review Process.* Department of Health, London.

14   Department of Health (2004) *NHS Job Evaluation Handbook* (2e). Department of Health, London.

15   Chambers R, Drinkwater C and Boath E (2002) *Involving Patients and the Public: how to do it better* (2e). Radcliffe Medical Press, Oxford.

16   Mohanna K and Chambers R (2000) *Risk Matters in Healthcare.* Radcliffe Medical Press, Oxford.

17   Hart E and Fletcher J (1999) Learning how to change: a selective analysis of literature and experience of how teams learn and organisations change. *Journal of Interprofessional Care.* **13(1)**: 53–63.

18   Maxwell RJ (1984) Quality assessment in health. *British Medical Journal.* **288**: 1470–2.

19   Firth-Cozens J (1993) *Audit in Mental Health Services.* LEA, Howe.

20   McCulloch D (2003) *Valuing Health in Practice.* Ashgate Publishing Ltd, Aldershot.

3

Demonstrating common components of good quality healthcare

In looking at the quality of care you provide and demonstrating your standards of service delivery and outcomes of learning, you should find that obtaining informed consent from patients for their treatment, maintaining confidentiality and handling complaints are part of the fabric of good quality care. We have considered them separately in this chapter, but each may be individualised to any of the five clinical areas of Chapters 4 to 8.

We have set out the chapter with key information about consent followed by some example cycles of the stages of evidence (*see* Figure 1.1 on page 6). The two other sections on confidentiality and complaints follow, laid out in similar ways. Read through the cycles of evidence to become familiar with the approach to gathering and documenting evidence of your learning, competence, performance or standards of service delivery. Then either adopt one of the examples or adapt it to your own circumstances. Alternatively, read on to one or more of the clinical chapters and look at these three components in a clinical context such as in relation to depression or dementia in Chapters 4 and 5.

Consent

Key points

Information given to a health professional remains the property of the patient. In most circumstances, consent is assumed for the necessary sharing of information with other professionals involved with the care of the patient for that episode of care. Usually consent is also assumed for essential sharing of information for continuing care. Beyond this, informed consent must be obtained. Patients attend for healthcare in the belief that the personal information that they supply, or which is found out about them during investigation or treatment, will be confidential. The NMC *Code of Professional Conduct* provides specific advice on protecting confidential information.[1]

Confidential information may be disclosed in the following circumstances:[1]

- if the patient consents
- if it is in the patient's own interest that information should be disclosed, but it is either impossible to seek the patient's consent or

- if it is medically undesirable in the patient's own interest, to seek the patient's consent
- if the law requires (and does not merely permit) the health professional to disclose the information
- if disclosure is needed for the interest of the public (e.g. in order to protect the patient from risk of harm)
- in issues of child protection, when you must act within local and national policies.

Health professionals must be able to justify their decision to disclose information without consent. If they are in any doubt, they should consult their professional bodies and colleagues.

Consent is only valid if the patient fully understands the nature and consequences of disclosure – they must be able to give their consent, receive enough information to enable them to make a decision and be acting under their own free will and not persuaded by the strong influence of another person. If consent is given, the health worker is responsible for limiting the disclosure to that information for which informed consent has been obtained. The development of modern information technology and the increasing amount of multidisciplinary teamwork in patient care make confidentiality difficult to uphold.

You may need to give information about a patient to a relative or carer. Normally the consent of the patient should be obtained. Sometimes, the clinical condition of the patient may prevent informed consent being obtained (e.g. they are unconscious or have a severe illness). It is important to recognise that relatives or carers do *not* have any right to information about the patient. Disclosure without consent may be justified when third parties are exposed to a risk so serious that it outweighs the patient's privacy. An example would be if a patient declines to allow you to disclose information about their health and continues to drive against medical advice when unfit to do so.

Local research ethics committees and the research governance framework ensure best practice in the giving of informed consent by patients in research studies.

As health professionals, we often assume implied consent. The general public and patients are generally ignorant of the extent to which information about them is passed around the NHS. We may incorrectly assume when teaching at both pre-registration and post-registration levels, in examinations and assessments and in research that patients imply their consent. Consent is also implied for health service accounting, central monitoring of referrals, in disease registers, for audit and in facilitating joint working between team members. The NHS is still engaged in a debate about what data can legitimately be shared without patients' explicit consent. Although written consent is usually obtained for supplying information to insurance companies or for legal reports, patients are often unaware of the type of information being supplied and may not have not given 'informed consent'.

Consent to treatment with medication is also often assumed – the doctor or nurse prescribes the medication and the patient takes it.[2] However, we know that a prescription may not be taken to the pharmacy for dispensing, or if it is, the medication is not started, or continued. You need to think about how you move from compliance to concordance as defined below:

- *compliance* with treatment or lifestyle changes implies that the patient follows instructions from health professionals to a greater or lesser degree

- *concordance* is a negotiated agreement on treatment between the patient and the healthcare professional. It allows patients to take informed decisions on the degree of risk or suffering that they themselves wish to undertake or follow.

Seeking consent is a fundamental part of good practice, and issues around validity and capacity to consent are covered in greater depth in the Department of Health reference guide or can be explored on the website.[3]

Collecting data to demonstrate your learning, competence, performance and standards of service delivery: consent

Example cycle of evidence 3.1

- Focus: informed consent
- Other relevant focus: research

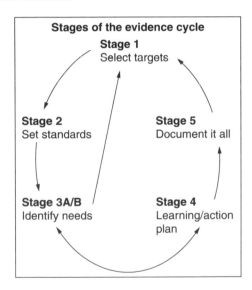

Stages of the evidence cycle

Stage 1
Select targets

Stage 2
Set standards

Stage 5
Document it all

Stage 3A/B
Identify needs

Stage 4
Learning/action plan

Case study 3.1

You agree as a practice to undertake a survey to find out if patients are satisfied with your service. The practice manager will organise it, but you are nominated to lead the work. You decide to focus on teenagers as a group as the adolescent drop-in clinic you set up two years ago with the school health service is not being used as much as it once was. You want to be proactive about helping teenagers resist smoking and drugs, encourage healthy eating and exercise, protect their mental health and encourage their management of chronic diseases such as asthma and diabetes, etc. You are not sure how to survey the teenagers. You think they are unlikely to answer questionnaires sent through the post and think you will interview teenagers about their satisfaction with the clinic. You intend to employ one of your own teenage children to interview some who have never come to the clinic, by selecting their names from your patient list as well as some teenagers who have attended. You're not sure if you are getting into research territory or if it is okay to claim you are auditing your services.

This is just an example. Keep your task simple. You could choose three or four cycles of evidence to demonstrate your competence each year.

Stage 1: Select your aspirations for good practice

The excellent nurse:

- protects patients' rights and makes sure that they are not disadvantaged by taking part in research
- gives patients the information they need about their problem in a way they can understand as a basis for informed consent.

Stage 2: Set the standards for your outcomes

Outcomes might include:
- the way learning is applied
- a learnt skill
- a protocol
- a strategy that is implemented
- meeting recommended standards.

- The informed consent policy of the practice covers patients' participation in audit and research as well as consent to clinical treatment.
- You are able to describe the difference between what is audit of clinical management and service provision and what is research.

Stage 3A: Identify your learning needs

- Read through the frequently asked questions and answers on the Department of Health website relating to research governance.[4] Consider whether you are able to answer the questions before reading the answers.
- Describe an audit plan of an adolescent clinic that involves obtaining young people's views of standards of services by interviewing them. Submit the plan to the chair of the local research ethics committee to check that he/she agrees that the audit proposal does not fall within the definition of research and to approve the patient literature and the process inviting informed consent to take part.
- Self-assess your own knowledge about teenagers consenting to treatment or research, and identify any differences in your approach if they are under or over the age of 16 years.

Stage 3B: Identify your service needs

Any of the needs assessment exercises in 3A may also reveal service needs.

- Draw up an information leaflet for young people about the audit of adolescent clinic services that you intend to carry out. Ask others to critique the leaflet – young people for its readability and clarity, a research colleague for the extent to which it conforms to best practice for informed consent. Use the information leaflet so that they can give informed consent to the interview to obtain their views and an audio recording of the interview.
- Ask a colleague to peer review the extent to which advice and information you give to teenagers during a consultation is accurate. The teenager would need to have given prior, written informed consent for the peer review (and audio-recording if used).

Stage 4: Make and carry out a learning and action plan

- Obtain and read the documents about research governance from the Department of Health's website or from your PCO – as in section 3A first point.[4]
- Study the application form for the ethical approval of a research study.
- Understand the limits to obtaining patients' views as part of audit of clinical and service management by reading up on informed consent. Look at whether you are explaining the details of the diagnosis or prognosis, and consider whether you routinely liaise with medical colleagues to discover what information they have given to patients. Consider whether you always give an explanation of likely benefits and side-effects of treatment, and what will happen if no treatment is given. Ensure that patients are always made to understand if proposed treatment is experimental and if students in training will be involved in their care.
- Ask for a short tutorial from your local clinical governance lead about good practice in obtaining patients' views through audit, research and patient involvement activities –

including good practice in informed consent and any special considerations for teenagers aged under 16 years.

Stage 5: Document your learning, competence, performance and standards of service delivery

- Keep a comparison of your own practice with the answers to the frequently asked questions on the Department of Health website relating to research governance.[4]
- File a copy of the response letter from the chair of local research ethics committee about the audit proposal.
- Document that the subsequent revised audit plan shows that the work does not fall within the definition of research.
- Keep a copy of the revised teenage patients' informed consent leaflet, following the critique.
- Repeat the peer review by the same, or another, colleague of the extent to which advice and information you give to teenagers during consultations is accurate.

Case study 3.1 continued

The chair of the research ethics committee advises you that your plan should be classed as research rather than audit as it involves contact with patients outside their usual NHS care. He explains about the risks of using untrained interviewers such as your own children, and the need to fully inform those teenagers you are inviting to be interviewed about the survey and that their refusal will not prejudice their medical care. He advises you to send an application form for formal approval to the ethics committee and to contact the research lead in your PCO in line with the research governance framework if you wish to continue to develop a research project. You revise your plans as the scale of the work required is becoming out of all proportion.

Confidentiality

Key points

You should have appropriate confidentiality safeguards in place in the practice to prevent inadvertent disclosure of personal and sensitive information about patients. Tell people, especially the young, about their right to confidential medical treatment and reinforce your conversation with posters and leaflets. People with non-prescription drug-related problems who seek help from substance abuse clinics, or those with sexually transmitted infections who attend genitourinary medicine clinics, often do not want their general practitioner (GP) surgery to be told because they do not believe that the information will be kept confidential. Fears about confidentiality are the commonest reason young people give for not attending their general practice surgery for contraceptive treatment.[5]

Young people under the age of 16 years have the same rights to confidentiality as other patients. The younger the person, the greater care is needed to assess the level of understanding to ensure that he or she understands the consequences of any proposed action. If a young person fulfils the conditions given in Box 3.1 he or she is regarded as being competent to make his or her own decisions.

Box 3.1:   The Fraser Guidelines[6]

The guidelines were drawn up after Lord Fraser stated in 1985 that a health professional could give contraceptive advice or treatment to a person under 16 years old without parental consent, providing that the professional is satisfied that:

- the young person will understand the advice
- the young person cannot be persuaded to tell their parents or allow the doctor to tell them that they are seeking contraceptive advice
- the young person is likely to begin or continue having unprotected sex with or without contraceptive treatment
- the young person's physical or mental health is likely to suffer unless they receive contraceptive advice or treatment
- it is in the young person's best interest to receive contraceptive advice or treatment.

The Fraser Guidelines apply to health professionals in England and Wales. In Scotland, the Age of Legal Capacity (Scotland) Act 1991 gives similar powers of consent to those under 16 years of age. In Northern Ireland, separate legislation applies. The Fraser Guidelines are included within the *Best Practice Guidance for Doctors and Other Health Professionals on the Provision of Advice and Treatment to Young People Under 16 on Contraception, Sexual and Reproductive Health* published by the Department of Health in July 2004.[6]

Occasionally you may feel that you have a moral obligation to divulge confidential information. Whenever possible you should seek to persuade the patient to give consent to the disclosure. Seek advice from your professional organisations in circumstances where others are at danger (e.g. risk of harm, or rape or sexual abuse), or where a serious crime has been committed. Health professionals should satisfy themselves that sufficient authority has been obtained (e.g. a certificate from the Attorney General or Lord Advocate) and consult professional organisations before disclosing information without a patient's consent.

The Caldicott Committee Report described principles of good practice to safeguard confidentiality when information is being used for non-clinical purposes:[7]

- justify the purpose
- do not use patient-identifiable information unless it is absolutely necessary
- use the minimum necessary patient-identifiable information
- access to patient-identifiable information should be on a strict need-to-know basis

- everyone with access to patient-identifiable information should be aware of his or her responsibilities.

Interpreters should be used wherever possible to avoid the use of friends or relatives. They should be trained in the requirements of confidentiality.

Patients are entitled to access data held about them. Exceptions to this right are:

- the patient failed to make the request in accordance with the Data Protection Act 1998
- if acceding to the request would result in disclosure of information about somebody else without their consent
- when giving medical information may cause serious harm to the mental or physical health of the patient (a rare occurrence).

You need to incorporate systems for ensuring that paper and computer security are maintained. Systems for monitoring and upgrading security systems should be in place and you should check regularly that confidentiality is not being breached if changes are made.

Collecting data to demonstrate your learning, competence, performance and standards of service delivery: confidentiality

Example cycle of evidence 3.2

- Focus: confidentiality
- Other relevant focus: teaching and training

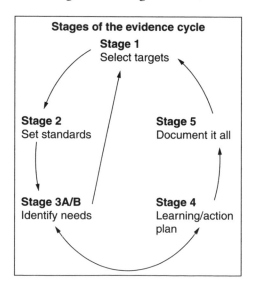

Stages of the evidence cycle

Stage 1
Select targets

Stage 2
Set standards

Stage 5
Document it all

Stage 3A/B
Identify needs

Stage 4
Learning/action plan

Case study 3.2

It is the first time you have had student nurses placed with you and you want to ensure that they are aware of the professional guidelines on confidentiality, and teach them about the importance of making sure that student visitors understand the practice code on confidentiality while they are on their placement with you.

This is just an example. Keep your task simple. You could choose three or four cycles of evidence to demonstrate your competence each year.

Stage 1: Select your aspirations for good practice

The excellent nurse:

- maintains the confidentiality of patient-specific information
- ensures that patients are aware of when they are receiving care from students and are not put at risk.

Stage 2: Set the standards for your outcomes

Outcomes might include:

- the way learning is applied
- a learnt skill
- a protocol
- a strategy that is implemented
- meeting recommended standards.

- Ensure that all members of the practice team, including you, new members of staff and students or others in training, are familiar with guidelines for confidentiality in relation to patients receiving healthcare.

Stage 3A: Identify your learning needs

- Assess your knowledge about the limits of confidentiality, e.g. for providing help for under-16 year olds with a drug problem or divulging information about the health of patients with cancer to relatives or carers.

- Ask an expert tutor's opinion about the particular method of teaching you plan to use for an in-house training session. The session will be on maintaining confidentiality for teenagers of different ages and people with life-threatening health problems. It should convey main messages and lead to changes where necessary.

Stage 3B: Identify your service needs

> Any of the needs assessment exercises in 3A may also reveal service needs.

- Compare the practice protocol for confidentiality with the guidelines in the *Confidentiality and Young People* toolkit.[5]
- Review your current or the intended induction programme for new members of staff, students on placement and doctors in training, to assess the extent to which knowledge of confidentiality features and is addressed.
- Organise a test of several different examples of patient episodes for members of the practice team, where confidentiality is complex and students or staff may be uncertain about the correct approach, based on the frequently asked questions on confidentiality published by the General Medical Council (GMC).[8,9]

Stage 4: Make and carry out a learning and action plan

- Find out from the local educational tutor how to undertake learning needs assessments of others from different disciplines with different levels of responsibilities in respect of confidentiality.
- Prepare for and run an interactive teaching session on confidentiality for patients of all age groups and conditions. You might invite the whole practice team, including students, family planning or school nurses, local pharmacists, GP registrars, etc. You could use the *Confidentiality and Young People* toolkit and the answers to the GMC's frequently asked questions, for promoting discussion with the practice team at the session.[5,9]

Stage 5: Document your learning, competence, performance and standards of service delivery

- Keep the answers of the quiz completed by those attending the teaching session before and after their training about confidentiality.
- Keep an incident record kept by the practice team of any reported or perceived breaches of confidentiality by anyone working in, or associated with, the practice.
- Include examples of personal learning plans based on learning needs assessments for new staff or doctors in training by the end of their induction period.
- Include the revised practice protocol in line with the *Confidentiality and Young People* toolkit and GMC guidance on confidentiality.[5,8]

Case study 3.2 continued

Other staff colleagues join your teaching session with the students using the video from the *Confidentiality and Young People* toolkit.[5] All get full marks in the quiz after watching the video. The frequently asked questions published by the GMC really enhance their understanding about how confidentiality issues are managed in practice.[9]

Learning from complaints

Key points

There is learning to be had from every complaint. Even if the complaint is trivial or undeserved it implies a lack of communication. Hence the basis of any complaints procedure should be about good communication. Complaints are often addressed defensively because of fear of criticism or litigation.[10] Poor communication is likely to generate misunderstandings and good communication can help to defuse difficult situations. Often the complainant is merely looking for an opportunity to give full expression to his concerns and to establish an opportunity to gain the full facts. Many complaints highlight failings in systems and processes which can be easily altered to prevent repetition of error.

Collecting data to demonstrate your learning, competence, performance and standards of service delivery: complaints

Example cycle of evidence 3.3

- Focus: complaints
- Other relevant focus: working with colleagues

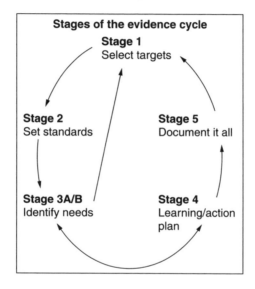

Stages of the evidence cycle

Stage 1
Select targets

Stage 2
Set standards

Stage 5
Document it all

Stage 3A/B
Identify needs

Stage 4
Learning/action plan

Case study 3.3

The practice where you work has received a patient complaint about lack of privacy for patients in the treatment room. This has prompted you all as a practice team to review the way that your complaints system functions.

This is just an example. Keep your task simple. You could choose three or four cycles of evidence to demonstrate your competence each year.

Stage 1: Select your aspirations for good practice

The excellent nurse:

- apologises appropriately when things go wrong, and has an adequate complaints procedure in place
- is not afraid of complaints, recognising that they can have positive outcomes of improving future ways of working.

Stage 2: Set the standards for your outcomes

Outcomes might include:

- the way learning is applied
- a learnt skill
- a protocol
- a strategy that is implemented
- meeting recommended standards.

- Understand and establish effective processes for preventing and managing complaints from patients in the practice.

Stage 3A: Identify your learning needs

- Examine as a significant event one or more complaints, e.g. where the practice has not advised a patient correctly about the complaints process.
- Compare the actual care of a patient against an acceptable standard of care for a range of clinical conditions as ongoing review for a clinical area that has been the subject of a complaint (e.g. privacy given to patients as in the case study). You could use peer review by asking respected colleagues, or compare your practice against a published standard such as a the *Essence of Care* privacy and dignity benchmark,[11] or a guideline by a responsible body of professional opinion.

Stage 3B: Identify your service needs

Any of the needs assessment exercises in 3A may also reveal service needs.

- Audit patient complaints in the preceding 12 months: the number, the outcomes and how the complaint system is advertised, etc.
- Audit the extent to which doctors and nurses are following practice-agreed protocols. Be proactive about preventing or minimising the likelihood of the source of the complaint recurring.

- Audit vulnerable areas. Look back at the analysis of complaints to identify useful areas for focusing learning, e.g. a review of the prescribing of steroids.
- Review the way that the qualifications of locums are checked and that they are made aware of the practice protocols.

Stage 4: Make and carry out a learning and action plan

- Ask your PCO to look at the practice complaints system and feed back how it can be improved (if at all).
- Arrange a tutorial between the practice manager and others in the team about preventing and managing complaints, or use one of the risk management packages produced by medical defence organisations.[12,13]
- Read up on how to undertake significant event analysis including how to share the information with the practice team and respond as a practice team.
- Score the *Essence of Care* privacy and dignity benchmark and share and compare as a practice team.[11]

Stage 5: Document your learning, competence, performance and standards of service delivery

- Include evidence of clinical competence to guard against a complaint.
- Include the protocol of the patient complaint process against which consecutive complaints can be audited in another 12 months' time.
- Record the guidance about physical examinations, including that the reason for any examination should be communicated clearly, that a chaperone should be offered for any internal or breast examination, and the comfort and privacy of the patient should always be kept in mind to avoid potential complaints.
- Record that a file containing practice protocols is available for easy reference on the desktop of the computer.
- Keep a record of benchmarking scores and action plans.

Case study 3.3 continued

You are invited by your PCO to take a lead in advising practices about the handling of complaints because they were impressed by the way your complaint system was applied when you discussed this in a meeting for community nurses.

References

1   Nursing and Midwifery Council (2002) *Code of Professional Conduct*. Nursing and Midwifery Council, London.

2   Chambers R and Wakley G (2000) *Making Clinical Governance Work for You*. Radcliffe Medical Press, Oxford.

3   Department of Health (2001) *Reference Guide to Consent for Examination and Treatment*. Department of Health, London. www.dh.gov.uk/assetRoot/04/01/90/79/04019079.pdf (accessed 26 April 2005)

4   www.dh.gov.uk/PolicyAndGuidance/ResearchAndDevelopment/fs/en (accessed 26 April 2005)

5   Royal College of General Practitioners and Brook (2000) *Confidentiality and Young People. A toolkit for general practice, primary care groups and trusts*. Royal College of General Practitioners, London.

6   www.dh.gov.uk/assetRoot/04/08/69/14/04086914.pdf (accessed 26 April 2005)

7   Department of Health (1997) Report of the review of patient-identifiable information. In: *The Caldicott Committee Report*. Department of Health, London.

8   General Medical Council (2004) *Confidentiality: protecting and providing information*. General Medical Council, London.

9   General Medical Council (2004) *Frequently Asked Questions. Confidentiality: protecting and providing information*. General Medical Council, London. *See* www.gmc-uk.org for updated questions and answers (accessed 26 April 2005)

10 Dimond B (1995) *Legal Aspects of Nursing*. Prentice Hall Nursing Series, London.

11 Department of Health (2003) *Essence of Care: patient-focused benchmarks for clinical governance*. NHS Modernisation Agency, London. Also *see* www.modern.nhs.uk (accessed 26 April 2005)

12 MPS Risk Consulting, Granary Wharf House, Leeds LS11 5PY or www.mps-riskconsulting.com (accessed 26 April 2005)

13 MDU Services Ltd, 230 Blackfriars Road, London SE1 8PJ or www.the-mdu.com (accessed 26 April 2005)

4

Depression

Nurses are now frequently taking a lead role in the management of chronic diseases and long-term conditions. Those who do take a lead role should be adequately qualified in that particular disease area to ensure the safety and quality of patient care. Qualifications can range from post-registration awards or certificates through to post-registration diplomas and degrees up to masters level. Competencies are gained through experience and supported by protocols. The multidisciplinary team approach in chronic disease management indicates that supplementary prescribing may be used for the management of long-term conditions and health needs. Supplementary prescribers must have a thorough knowledge of the area they prescribe in and of drugs and drug interactions, a clear management plan agreed with the independent prescriber and the patient, and be aware of their own limitations.

In a general practice surgery, every third or fourth patient seen has some form of mental disorder. There are greater levels of disability among primary care patients from mental disorders than from common chronic diseases such as hypertension, diabetes, arthritis and back pain. Good mental healthcare is a collaborative effort. The primary care team includes practice nurses, district nurses, health visitors, community psychiatric nurses, counsellors, clinical psychologists and school nurses as well as GPs, all of whom may have a role in mental healthcare.[1]

Episodes of 'major' depression are twice as common in women as men. Major depression is strongly associated with adverse life and economic circumstances – such as unemployment, divorce or poor housing. Depression is the most common mental health problem in older people, especially in those living in nursing and residential care: 10–15% of older adults, aged over 65 years, have significant depressive symptoms, although major depression is rare. Women are more likely to be depressed than men. Depressive symptoms are the fourth most important cause of disability worldwide. In the UK:

- about 90% of mental healthcare is delivered solely in primary care[2]
- depression accounts for 10% of all new diagnoses in primary care[3]
- antidepressant drugs account for 7% of UK primary care drug expenditure[3]
- untreated depressed patients use two to three times the annual medical services compared to their non-depressed counterparts[4]
- depression is a stronger predictor of serious cardiac disease during the year following cardiac catheterisation than smoking, severity of coronary artery disease and diminished left ventricular ejection fraction.[5]

It is generally held that GPs fail to diagnose up to half of cases of depression or anxiety. However, longitudinal studies have shown that most patients who did not receive a diagnosis of depression at a single consultation were given a diagnosis at subsequent consultations, or recovered without a GP's diagnosis.[6] GPs seem least likely to miss severe episodes of major depression – much of what is missed is mild and likely to improve spontaneously. Common triggers of depression are due to:

- psychological impact from major life events
- illnesses such as infectious diseases, hepatitis and influenza
- medications such as antihypertensives, oral contraceptives and corticosteroids
- others such as family history, childbirth, menopause, seasonal changes and chronic medical conditions.

Depression or other mental ill-health should not be considered as a stand-alone diagnosis. It often co-exists with physical, emotional and social problems and other psychiatric disorders such as alcohol and drug misuse, anxiety, obsessive–compulsive disorders and eating disorders.[7–10] Along with assessing for common mental health problems, equal emphasis should be placed on the approach and attitude practitioners use in their contact with patients. It is important to look at the whole person rather than focusing on a set of symptoms, and to consider the social and psychological aspects of the person's life.[1]

One study of frequent attenders to general practice found that depressive symptoms were the major predictor of frequent attendance rather than physical health problems.[11]

Case study 4.1

You recognise Mrs Down as she enters your consulting room. You know that, in the past, she suffered from two episodes of depression requiring treatment with antidepressants. Looking at her records, you see that she took tricyclic antidepressants for three months for both episodes. The last episode was about two years ago. She looks gloomy as she sits down and in response to your usual opening of 'How are you today?' promptly bursts into tears.

What issues you should cover[12–14]

Depression affects the majority of people at some time – so Mrs Down is in good company. Around 60–70% of adults will experience depression or worry of sufficient severity to influence their daily activities at some time in their lives.[12–14] Episodes of depression are short-lived for most people. Depression does not mean weakness, nor does it mean laziness. But it does mean that Mrs Down has a medical disorder that requires treatment. The primary care nurse needs to ensure a healthcare professional trained in the assessment and treatment of depression has assessed Mrs Down and discuss concerns with the GP.

Depression is one of the most common reasons for consulting a GP. Up to 50% of people attending general practice may have some depressive symptoms, of whom 5–10% have 'major' depression (*see* Box 4.1). The majority of people with depression are treated and managed in primary care. For a GP with an average list size of 1800 patients, there will be 111 working age adults with depression and/or anxiety warranting treatment and 40 older people with depression.

Symptoms and signs of depression[12]

Symptoms are summarised in Box 4.1. Depression and anxiety often present together. Physical symptoms may be the presenting feature(s) of depression and lead to delayed or missed diagnoses of depression. Several times as many people have one or some depressive symptoms as meet the criteria for major depression.[13]

Box 4.1: Criteria for 'major' depression[12]

At least five of the symptoms listed below must be present most of the day or nearly every day, during a two-week period, of which at least one must be 'depressed mood' or 'diminished interest or pleasure':

- depressed mood
- markedly diminished interest or pleasure in normal activities
- significant weight loss or gain
- insomnia or hypersomnia
- agitated or retarded
- fatigue or loss of energy
- feelings of worthlessness or excessive guilt
- diminished ability to think or concentrate, or indecisiveness
- recurrent thoughts of death or suicidal thoughts or actions.

The presentation of depression in people aged over 65 years may be atypical with low mood being masked. The patient may present with anxiety or memory impairment. The symptoms may be due to dementia, as depression and dementia commonly co-exist.

Depression may be 'bipolar' or 'unipolar'. The term 'bipolar' describes depression that occurs in conjunction with manic episodes. Other depression is termed 'unipolar' – as Box 4.2 describes.

Box 4.2: Classification of primary depression

Unipolar

- Single depressive episode:
    - mild, moderate or severe
    - with or without somatic syndrome
    - if severe, with or without psychotic symptoms
- Mixed anxiety and depressive disorder
- Recurrent depressive disorder
- Brief recurrent depression

- Seasonal affective disorder
- Dysthymia: depression intermittently for more than two years that does not fulfil criteria for mild or moderate depressive episode

Bipolar

- Bipolar affective disorder
- Cyclothymia: persistent instability of mood

Course of the illness[13]

About half the people who have major depression experience a further depressive episode in the following 10 years.

- *Mild to moderate depression*: sufferers have depressive symptoms and some functional impairment. Many recover in the short term, and about half have recurrent symptoms.
- *Severe depression*: sufferers have depressive symptoms plus agitation or psychomotor retardation and somatic symptoms. Common unexplained somatic complaints can include: headaches, chest pains, difficulty in breathing, difficulty in swallowing, nausea, vomiting, abdominal pain, lower back pain, skin rashes, frequent urination, diarrhoea, skin and muscle discomfort.
- *Psychotic depression*: sufferers have hallucinations, delusions or both in addition to their depressive symptoms.

Case study 4.1 continued

Mrs Down fits with the category mild to moderate depression, and you explain how common it is for depression to recur. She tells you that her brother committed suicide about 10 years previously and she confides that she dreads becoming so depressed that she does the same. You ascertain that although she is depressed she is not having suicidal thoughts.

Suicide and self-harm

Suicide rates are higher in people with depression; it has been estimated that 40–50% of all suicides are committed by people with undiagnosed or inadequately treated depressive disorders.[12] Suicides account for just under 1% of all deaths, of which nearly two-thirds occur in depressed people.[15] Box 4.3 describes the plans in the National Service Framework (NSF) for Mental Health, for preventing suicide; the concepts are generalisable throughout the UK.

Box 4.3: The approach to preventing suicide via the National Service Framework for England[16]

Local health and social care communities should prevent suicides by:

- *Standard one*: promoting mental health for all, working with individuals and communities
- *Standard two*: delivering high quality primary mental healthcare
- *Standard three:* ensuring that anyone with a mental health problem can contact local services via the primary care team, a helpline or an emergency department
- *Standard four:* ensuring that individuals with severe and enduring mental illness have a care plan which meets their specific needs, including access to services round the clock
- *Standard five:* providing safe hospital accommodation for individuals who need it
- *Standard six:* enabling individuals caring for someone with severe mental illness to receive the support that they need to continue to care
- *Standard seven:* in addition to the above:
  - supporting local prison staff in preventing suicides among prisoners
  - ensuring that staff are competent to assess the risk of suicide among individuals at greatest risk
  - developing local systems for suicide to learn lessons and take any necessary action.

Deliberate self-harm involves intentional self-poisoning or injury. It is one of the top five causes of acute medical admissions for both women and men in the UK. Around 50–60% of patients have visited their GP in the month before the episode of their self-harm.[17]

Risk factors for suicide include: unemployment, low income, being single and a history of mental illness necessitating hospital admission. High-risk groups include: the mentally ill, those with a history of parasuicide, alcoholics, prisoners and certain occupational groups such as doctors, pharmacists, farmers and vets. Methods used to commit suicide include overdose (24%), hanging (20%) and car exhaust fumes (20%).[15]

The target for year 2010 in England is to reduce the death rate from suicide and undetermined injury by at least a fifth – saving 4000 lives.[16]

Recommendations for psychiatric referral

Referral to psychiatric services is indicated:

- if there is a risk of suicide
- for psychotic symptoms
- with a history of a bipolar affective disorder

- when the practitioner feels insufficiently experienced to manage a patient's condition
- if two or more attempts to treat the patient's depressive disorder have failed or resulted in only partial response.

Case study 4.1 continued

Mrs Down asks you if she can try something different this time to 'cure' her depression as the last lot of antidepressants prescribed by the GP do not seem to have worked since her depression is back again. You explain to Mrs Down that she did not complete either of the previous two courses of antidepressants, as she did not return to consult you once she started to feel better and stopped taking her prescribed treatment. You therefore advise her to try a full course of antidepressant drugs this time, continuing with the treatment for at least four to six months after she starts to feel better, and consulting you or the GP regularly over that period.

Treatment of depressive disorders

You discuss with Mrs Down that there are two main approaches to treating depression:

1 psychological treatment (counselling or cognitive behavioural therapy)
2 medical treatment with antidepressant drugs.

Both therapies are most often needed – the supportive therapy for stress/life problems, patterns of negative thinking, and prevention of further episodes. The medication is needed for depressed mood or loss of interest/pleasure for two or more weeks and at least four of the symptoms shown in Box 4.1; for little response to supportive therapy (counselling); for recurrent depression; and for a family history of depression.[1]

Psychological treatments may be sufficient for mild forms of depression. For moderate or severe depression, antidepressants alone or in combination with psychological treatments may be appropriate. The evidence for the different approaches in the treatment of depressive disorders that are effective or likely to be beneficial is outlined in Box 4.4.

Box 4.4:   Effective interventions for depression[13,18,19]

- *Medication*:
    - tricyclic and heterocyclic antidepressants (in mild, moderate and severe depression)
    - monoamine oxidase inhibitors (in mild, moderate and severe depression)
    - selective serotonin reuptake inhibitors (SSRIs) and related drugs (in mild, moderate and severe depression)
    - St John's Wort (in mild to moderate depression)

- continuation treatment with antidepressant drugs (reduces risk of relapse in mild to moderate depression)
- *Psychotherapy*:
  - cognitive therapy (in mild to moderate depression)
  - interpersonal therapy (in mild to moderate depression)
  - problem-solving therapy (in mild to moderate depression)
- *Combined medication and psychotherapy* (in mild, moderate and severe depression)
- *Electroconvulsive therapy* (in severe depression)
- *Other approaches*:
  - care pathways (in mild to moderate depression)

There is a vast array of antidepressants available, and while a great deal of evidence exists for the effectiveness of SSRIs and tricyclic antidepressants, there is less evidence for the effectiveness of other neurotransmitter drugs. These others include drugs chemically related to, but different from, the tricyclic antidepressants such as trazodone and a range of other chemically unrelated antidepressants including mirtazapine. Other drugs used either alone or in combination with antidepressant drugs include lithium salts and the antipsychotics, although use of these drugs is usually reserved for people with severe, psychotic or chronic depression.[15]

The choice of antidepressant will be based on the individual person's requirements, including the presence of co-existing disease, current therapy, suicide risk and previous response to antidepressant medication. For instance, tricyclic drugs should be prescribed with special caution in people with epilepsy (as they lower the convulsive threshold) or with cardiac disease (as occasionally arrhythmias and heart block may occur); and one of the SSRI antidepressants which do not interact with alcohol should be chosen if the patient is unwilling to give up alcohol.

Lithium should only be prescribed by a specialist. The potential risks and benefits should be carefully weighed and the need for continued therapy regularly re-assessed. The primary care team should monitor the dose carefully because of the narrow therapeutic range and potential toxicity. The primary care team should monitor lithium levels every three months. The practice protocol for the management of lithium should be set up to recall patients every three months, so that blood tests can be arranged 12 hours post-dose. Serum creatinine and thyroid-stimulating hormone (TSH) should be checked every 6–12 months, as hypothyroidism and abnormal renal function are relatively common side-effects. Other problems that can arise include blurred vision, vomiting, dysarthria, ataxia, coarse tremor, reduced sex drive, drowsiness, confusion, seizures, coma and hypotension. Patients should be warned not to stop lithium abruptly, to avoid a rebound psychosis.

Figure 4.1 describes current guidelines for managing depression in primary care, updated by the British Association of Psychopharmacology (BAP).[18] These guidelines emphasise the importance of choosing an antidepressant drug that best suits the individual patient. There are several national clinical practice guidelines for depressive disorders. A review of such guidelines found 15, of which the BAP guidelines are one.[20]

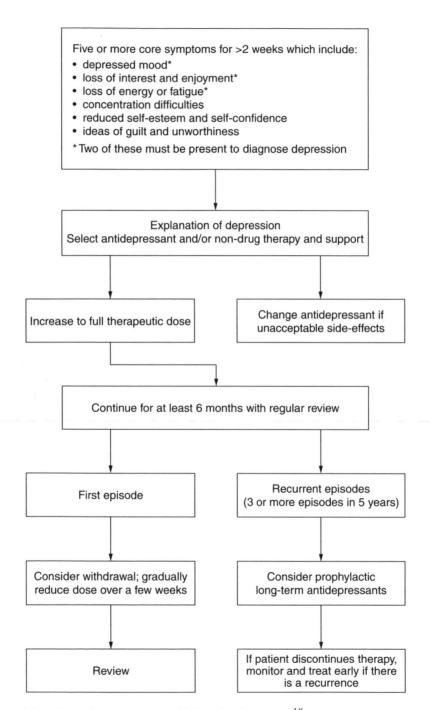

Figure 4.1: Current management guidelines for depression.[18]

SSRIs or tricyclic antidepressants are more effective than placebo in the treatment of major and minor depressive disorders.[13] Antidepressants are more effective than placebo in the treatment of chronic mild depressive disorders.[13,16]

When SSRIs are compared with tricyclic antidepressants in people with all grades of depression there is no clinically significant difference in effectiveness.[13,21] Research comparing side-effects of SSRIs and tricyclics found that tricyclic antidepressants were associated with higher rates of adverse effects, but the difference was small.[13] Abrupt withdrawal of SSRIs is associated with symptoms such as dizziness, nausea, paraesthesia, headache and vertigo.[13]

Monoamine oxidase inhibitors (MAOIs) are occasionally used as second-line drugs and must be used with caution because of the potential serious adverse effect of a hypertensive crisis occurring without dietary limitation. Compared with tricyclic drugs, MAOIs are less effective in treating severe depressive disorders, but more effective in treating atypical depressive disorders, characterised by increased sleep, increased appetite, mood reactivity, and rejection sensitivity.[13]

Antidepressant medication is highly effective when used properly, but depression is often inadequately treated and depressed patients may receive either no medication or sub-therapeutic doses of medication – as in Mrs Down's case.[22]

The array of clinical practice guidelines that exist for depression focus mainly on major depression, rather than the mild to moderate depression that is commonly seen in primary care. This does limit their applicability and relevance to those working in primary care and the types of patients being treated in primary, as opposed to secondary care.

Case study 4.1 continued

You work hard to inform Mrs Down about the rationale for treating depression with medication, and the benefits and risks of treatments, to gain her concordance. You discuss the dose and different types of antidepressant drugs and the possibility of continuing medication to prevent a future return of her depression. After your discussion Mrs Down feels that she could make an informed choice and elects to try an SSRI, which might have fewer side-effects than the tricyclic drug she had taken before, and you agree to meet monthly. You discuss the possibility of starting cognitive therapy as well as taking the medication, to help to prevent relapse.

Prescribing tips

From compliance to concordance

Research has shown that up to 8% of prescriptions for antidepressants are never dispensed.[23] Many drugs that are dispensed are not consumed. At least 25–50% of patients on antidepressant medication take irregular or insufficient doses. So you should find ways to encourage patients to adhere to the drugs prescribed, by giving them better information so that they can take part in the decision to take antidepressants and be more likely to 'own' that agreement. Understanding the differences between compliance and concordance may help nurses and doctors to structure a negotiated agreement rather than issue instructions to the patient. Supplementary prescribers will agree a clinical management plan (CMP) between the supplementary prescriber, the independent prescriber and the patient.

In the past, the term 'non-compliance' was used to highlight the situation when many patients were unable or unwilling to take their medication as prescribed. However, the term 'non-compliance' portrays the unequal partnership between patients and health professionals. Implicit in the term 'compliance' is the idea that patients take orders from health professionals.

Concordance describes a two-way communication that recognises that the health beliefs of the patient, although different from those of nurse, doctor or pharmacist, are no less valuable or important in deciding the best approach to the treatment of the individual. Concordance is a therapeutic partnership reached between the patient and the healthcare professional following negotiation, that respects the beliefs and wishes of the patient even if that means that he/she decides not to take their medicine or to alter their treatment in some way.[24]

Keep dosing schedules as simple as possible to aid concordance. Patients should be counselled that it usually takes at least two weeks for them to notice any benefit from antidepressants.[19]

Dose

SSRI drugs can be started at the recommended maintenance dose except in the elderly where it is wise to start with half the normal adult dose and titrate upwards as necessary to gain clinical improvement. As most side-effects vary with dose, gradually increase the dose until side-effects appear and then slowly decrease the dose until they disappear or are tolerable.[24]

MAOIs should not be prescribed within six weeks of discontinuing fluoxetine because of its long half-life, within two weeks of paroxetine, mirtazapine and sertraline, or within one week of citalopram, fluvoxamine and venlafaxine.

Dependence and withdrawal

Reassure patients that antidepressants are not addictive. Once an antidepressant has been taken for more than a few weeks, there should be at least a planned four-week tapering off period when they are discontinued to avoid any reaction. The abrupt withdrawal of SSRIs such as paroxetine and fluvoxamine, which have a short half-life, can lead to a 'discontinuation syndrome' in up to one in five patients. This is characterised by transient flu-like symptoms including dizziness, nausea, paraesthesia, headache, tremor, palpitations, vertigo and anxiety.[13] Withdrawal reactions have been reported more frequently for paroxetine than for sertraline and fluoxetine.[13]

Continuation and maintenance treatment

Continuing treatment with antidepressant drugs for 4–6 months after recovery (in mild or moderate depression) reduces the risk of relapse by almost half; for the elderly this period should be extended to 12 months.[13]

Reinforce that long-term treatment for recurrent depressive disorder should be maintained, in order to prevent the recurrence of further depressive episodes. Several trials have found that maintenance treatment reduces the relapse rate in recurrent depressive disorder compared with placebo.[13]

Consider maintenance or prophylactic treatment with antidepressant drugs for people who have had three or more recent episodes of significant depression or more than five episodes altogether.

Other treatments

Electroconvulsive therapy

Electroconvulsive therapy (ECT) is effective in treating patients with acute severe depressive disorder.[13] ECT is a short-term treatment that may be useful when a rapid response is required. People often complain of memory impairment following ECT. This treatment should be reserved for those who cannot tolerate drugs or who have not responded to other treatment, where a rapid response is required in severe depression considered to be life-threatening or in catatonia, or a prolonged or severe manic episode.[25]

Specific psychological treatments

Interpersonal psychotherapy, problem-solving therapy and non-directive counselling have been found to be as effective as drugs in treating mild to moderate depression in people of all ages.[13]

Cognitive behavioural therapy

This is a 'talking' therapy used for people suffering from depression, anxiety and eating disorders.[13] In cognitive behavioural therapy (CBT), links are made between the person's feelings and patterns of thinking that underpin their distress. The patient is encouraged to take an active part in examining the evidence for and against distressing beliefs, challenging the habitual patterns of thinking about the belief and using reasoning and personal experience to develop rational and acceptable alternatives. Therapy may typically be carried out as 20 sessions over 12 to 16 weeks with some occasional follow-up booster sessions.[13] It is provided by clinical psychologists, psychiatrists or community psychiatric nurses.

Cognitive therapy focuses on changing the dysfunctional beliefs and negative automatic thoughts that characterise depressive disorders. One review of published research demonstrated that cognitive therapy may be more effective than drug treatment in people with mild to moderate depression.[13]

Interpersonal psychotherapy

Interpersonal therapy (IPT) is a brief, standardised treatment for depression, which usually consists of 12–16 weekly sessions.[13] IPT is primarily used for people with unipolar non-psychotic depressive disorders. The therapeutic techniques employed focus on improving the patient's interpersonal functioning within current relationships and identifying the problems associated with the onset of the depressive episode in order to prevent relapse. Patients are initially educated about the nature of depression and reassured that their various symptoms are part of their depression. The depressive symptoms are addressed in a similar fashion to the behavioural techniques used in cognitive behavioural therapy. The therapist then moves on to address the interpersonal issues relevant for that individual. The main problem areas are then defined and become the focus of therapy.[19]

Problem solving

Problem solving is briefer and simpler than cognitive therapy and so may be feasible within a primary care setting.[13] It consists of three stages:

1 identifying the main problems for the patient
2 generating solutions
3 trying out the solutions.

Non-directive counselling

This was developed by Rogers in 1961 and aims to help people to express feelings and to clarify thoughts and difficulties.[26] The therapist does not give direct advice, but suggests alternative understandings and encourages people to solve their own problems.

St John's Wort (hypericum perforatum)

St John's Wort is more effective than placebo in the treatment of mild to moderate depressive disorders, and is as effective as prescription antidepressant drugs. However, this evidence must be interpreted with caution as the research upon which this report is based was not undertaken on fully representative groups of people using standardised preparations, and doses of antidepressants varied.[13,27] Hypericum is the active agent and may cause interactions with prescribed drugs.[28]

Acupuncture

Acupuncture may relieve depressive symptoms. Three Chinese trials indicated that acupuncture was as effective as tricyclic antidepressant drugs in relieving depression.[27]

Exercise

There is limited evidence that exercise, alone or combined with other treatments, is beneficial in mild to moderate depression.[13]

Screening for depression

None of the definitions and scores that can categorise depression are used routinely in primary care.[29] Research suggests that most depression that is treated in primary care is below, or just reaches, the minimum diagnostic criteria for major depression (*see* Box 4.1). GPs appear to see their patients in terms of 'fluctuating mood disturbances' occurring in response to life situations, often against the background of chronic difficulties, physical illness, insecure relationships and deprivation.[29]

Validated screening questionnaires cannot be recommended for systematic screening. They tend to be used in research on depression in primary care but there is no convincing evidence that identifying cases via validated questionnaires such as the Beck Depression Inventory or the Geriatric Depression Scale, or the Edinburgh Postnatal Depression tool improves clinical outcomes.[30,31] The presence of depression should be confirmed by clinical assessment of the state of the person's mental health. Although these screening tools may be used as an aide-mémoire, they do not replace professional judgement.

Quality and outcomes framework indicators in mental health[32]

Depression is a chronic disease that requires quality management as an essential service of general practice. This includes relevant health promotion, treatment and referral. Mental health is one of the 10 domains of chronic disease management specified within the General Medical Services (GMS) contract. Table 4.1 lists the quality indicators relevant to mental health and associated points. People with 'severe long-term mental health problems' are described in the NSF as 'patients who are managed by the care plan approach'.[16] These may include patients:

- suffering from severe or recurrent depression
- suffering from bipolar depression
- with a history of psychosis
- with drug and/or alcohol addiction.

It is not explicit whether all primary care organisations (PCOs) will include severe and enduring depression within the umbrella of 'severe long-term mental health problems' or will assume the term mainly applies to schizophrenia.

Table 4.1:   Quality indicators in mental health

Indicator		Points	Maximum threshold (%)
MH1	The practice can produce a register of people with severe long-term mental health problems who require and have agreed to regular follow-up	7	
MH2	The percentage of patients with severe long-term mental health problems with a review recorded in the preceding 15 months. This review includes a check on the accuracy of prescribed medication, a review of physical health and a review of co-ordination arrangements with secondary care	23	90
MH3	The percentage of patients on lithium therapy with a record of lithium levels checked within the previous 6 months	3	90
MH4	The percentage of patients on lithium therapy with a record of serum creatinine and TSH in the preceding 15 months	3	90
MH5	The percentage of patients on lithium therapy with a record of lithium levels in the therapeutic range within the previous 6 months	5	70

All minimum thresholds are 25%

Practices may contract to provide enhanced services covering the specialised care of depression. These practices should be able to:

• produce and maintain an up-to-date register of depressed patients
• apply a multidisciplinary approach
• use cognitive behavioural therapy
• use screening procedures
• undertake appropriate training
• maintain personal health plans
• make referrals and inquiries as clinically indicated
• perform an annual review
• receive feedback from patients and their families using an appropriate questionnaire.

Collecting data to demonstrate your learning, competence, performance and standards of service delivery

Example cycle of evidence 4.1

- Focus: clinical care – depression
- Other relevant foci: relationships with patients; working with colleagues

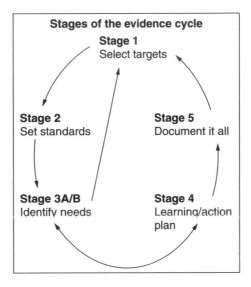

Stages of the evidence cycle

Stage 1
Select targets

Stage 2
Set standards

Stage 5
Document it all

Stage 3A/B
Identify needs

Stage 4
Learning/action plan

Case study 4.2

Ms Sadd comes to see you, her health visitor, cuddling her nine-month-old baby to her in a sling. She sits down and bursts into tears. She is finding it increasingly difficult to get through her work in the local tourist information service and look after her son, as she is so tired. Her partner works away from home so she feels like a single parent, always being the one to take and collect her son from nursery and look after him when he's sick. Her work is suffering and she was disciplined last week for losing her temper with customers. She asks if she should ask her GP for for tablets to help her to sleep better so that she can cope with work and as a mum.

This is just an example. Keep your task simple. You could choose three or four cycles of evidence to demonstrate your competence each year.

Stage 1: Select your aspirations for good practice

The excellent health visitor:

- takes time to elicit all relevant details of a patient's history
- explains the diagnosis to a patient so that they can make an informed choice about treatment and management options.

Stage 2: Set the standards for your outcomes

Outcomes might include:

- the way learning is applied
- a learnt skill
- a protocol
- a strategy that is implemented
- meeting recommended standards.

- Agree a practice protocol with health visitor colleagues and GPs for managing women with postnatal depression.
- Map out the local support services available to women with postnatal depression.

Stage 3A: Identify your learning needs

- Self-assess whether you are up to date with treatment of postnatal depression.
- Carry out a significant event audit of a patient who was diagnosed with postnatal depression by another health visitor when the baby was one year old. You had seen the patient for feeding problems and you realise looking back that the patient had postnatal depression for many months.

Stage 3B: Identify your service needs

Any of the needs assessment exercises in 3A may also reveal service needs.

- Discuss the findings of the significant event audit in 3A (second point) as a team at an educational meeting in the practice. Check whether all members of team are aware of services available to women with postnatal depression, e.g. benefit payments, psychological therapies, Sure Start, Home Start, childcare centres etc.
- Audit the extent to which women who have been treated for postnatal depression in the previous 12 months have been followed up by the team or by an individual health visitor.

Stage 4: Make and carry out a learning and action plan

- Arrange a tutorial with a health visitor with a special interest in postnatal depression, to include the use of a screening questionnaire.
- Read an interesting paper in a nursing journal.[33]
- Run an educational session in the practice where you present best practice guidance for managing postnatal depression after reading up on the topic and the tutorial with a health visitor. You present a draft protocol for managing postnatal depression, which those present discuss and agree. The session culminates by the team pooling their knowledge to map out the support services available for women with postnatal depression.

Stage 5: Document your learning, competence, performance and standards of service delivery

- Draw a flow diagram of the services available to women with postnatal depression.
- Include the updated and agreed practice protocol for managing postnatal depression.
- Audit the extent of the follow-up for patients with postnatal depression, including the proportion who start on medication who continue on medication for at least six months. Include any necessary action plan.
- Record the discussions and conclusions from the significant event audit of the delay in recognition of postnatal depression and the reasons for the delayed diagnosis.

Case study 4.2 continued

Ms Sadd accepts your diagnosis of depression. She considers the options of no treatment, taking antidepressant tablets and/or seeing a community psychiatric nurse for counselling, and opts for antidepressant medication. She prefers to continue at work and not take sickness leave. You go round to see Ms Sadd at home on her day off work and your discussion and advice help Ms Sadd to understand her feelings and make a practical plan with her partner to relieve some of the pressure she is under from working almost full-time and acting as a single parent.

Example cycle of evidence 4.2

- Focus: good nursing practice
- Other relevant foci: confidentiality; consent

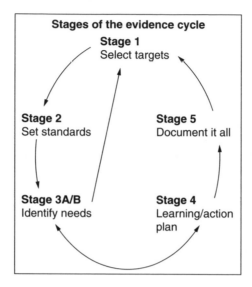

Stages of the evidence cycle

Stage 1
Select targets

Stage 2
Set standards

Stage 5
Document it all

Stage 3A/B
Identify needs

Stage 4
Learning/action plan

Case study 4.3

Following a bereavement visit to Mrs Lowe, her son Jack arrives as you, the district nurse, are just about to get in your car and return to the surgery. He explains that he lives 10 miles from his mother, and sees her about once a month. She rarely goes out and he is worried that she is not eating and is losing weight and often smells as if she's been drinking sherry. She used to be house proud but her house is now untidy and she just does not seem to care about the mess. Since her husband died, she's become more and more of a recluse. He doesn't feel he can do any more as she just asks tearfully to be left alone.

This is just an example. Keep your task simple. You could choose three or four cycles of evidence to demonstrate your competence each year.

Stage 1: Select your aspirations for good practice

The excellent nurse:

- is sure about the limits of confidentiality when talking to a person about another patient without their explicit permission
- provides proactive care to patients suffering from depression.

Stage 2: Set the standards for your outcomes

Outcomes might include:

- the way learning is applied
- a learnt skill
- a protocol
- a strategy that is implemented
- meeting recommended standards.

- Develop a protocol for bereavement visiting, recognising when the normal bereavement process has become clinical depression.
- Nurses will have the skills to detect and respond to mental health problems.

Stage 3A: Identify your learning needs

- Keep a reflective diary noting down your suspicions of co-existing mental ill-health as you visit your elderly patients. Compare your reflections with what is revealed at successive consultations with you or your colleagues.
- Invite feedback from colleagues about whether your care of elderly patients is appropriate, e.g. from district nursing colleagues, GPs, health visitors, receptionists.
- Review how you would or could recognise depression with the community psychiatric nurse. Invite her to comment on gaps in your knowledge.

Stage 3B: Identify your service needs

Any of the needs assessment exercises in 3A may also reveal service needs.

- Carry out a significant event audit arising from a breach of confidentiality relating to one of the practice team giving out patient-specific information to a relative without explicit consent from the patient concerned.

Stage 4: Make and carry out a learning and action plan

- Continue the discussion of the gaps with the community psychiatric nurse with a tutorial on best practice in managing depression, especially alternative approaches to medication.
- Contact local voluntary bereavement services or your local hospice for advice on protocols/guidelines for bereavement visiting.
- Read up on care pathways for mild to moderate depression. Get involved with the primary care organisation (PCO) mental health local implementation team (LIT) to discuss composing a care pathway.
- Phone the PCO Caldicott guardian to discuss problems and issues with confidentiality of patient information where it is difficult to assess the fitness or competence of patients to make decisions about their care (e.g. those with signs of senility, those inebriated, children).

Stage 5: Document your learning, competence, performance and standards of service delivery

- Keep a copy of your draft care pathway.
- Include a copy of the guidance notes for the practice team on handling patient confidentiality where there are complicating issues.
- Include a copy of the bereavement visiting protocol.
- Extract anonymised comments from your reflective diary and your planned developments.

Case study 4.3 continued

You explain that you are not able to discuss an able patient with anyone else, including a close relative, without their permission, but you are willing to listen to Jack's concerns about Mrs Lowe and to take what action you consider appropriate. You realise that Mrs Lowe may be at risk from her seeming depression and alcohol misuse and discuss this with the GP and CPN. You are able to chat with Mrs Lowe about her loneliness, isolation and depression and agree with her that she will attend the surgery to consult with the GP about her depression, and you arrange for social services to review her social care needs.

Example cycle of evidence 4.3

- Focus: working with colleagues
- Other relevant focus: health and safety

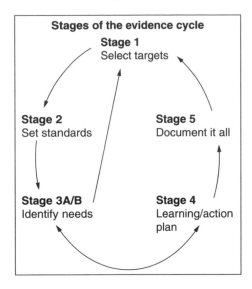

Stages of the evidence cycle

Stage 1
Select targets

Stage 2
Set standards

Stage 5
Document it all

Stage 3A/B
Identify needs

Stage 4
Learning/action
plan

Case study 4.4

Mrs Burden is qualified as a supplementary prescriber in her practice nurse role within the practice. Unfortunately she is going through a bad patch at present at home – her mother has a terminal illness, one of her children has been suspended from school and she is recently divorced. She puts a brave face on at work and none of the staff realise that she is depressed. They know that she is forgetful, is rude to patients, makes mistakes in the doses of drugs she is prescribing and takes much longer to do jobs than she used to. The practice manager talks about Mrs Burden's manner at work with you as the senior nurse who leads on nursing matters, and you both realise that all your concerns relate to the last year – before that Mrs Burden had a different approach to work and you were all pleased with the standards of her work. You offer to chat with her to find out if there's anything going on to account for her changed attitude to work.

> This is just an example. Keep your task simple. You could choose three or four cycles of evidence to demonstrate your competence each year.

Stage 1: Select your aspirations for good practice

The excellent nurse:

- is interested in and concerned about the health and wellbeing of colleagues at work
- recognises when ill-health factors affect a colleague's work and takes appropriate action.

Stage 2: Set the standards for your outcomes

Outcomes might include:

- the way learning is applied
- a learnt skill
- a protocol
- a strategy that is implemented
- meeting recommended standards.

- The practice policy on health and wellbeing is copied to all practice team members. It describes primary care team members' responsibilities and what action to take when patient safety is at risk.

Stage 3A: Identify your learning needs

- Recall if there has been any similar incident in the past when you feared that a member of staff was under-performing in a way that put patient safety at risk. Identify what action you or others took. Consider if the action was appropriate, could have been improved or a more prompt response made.
- Discuss the nature of an employer's responsibility for under-performing staff with the practice manager, who worked previously as a manager in industry in charge of many staff.

Stage 3B: Identify your service needs

Any of the needs assessment exercises in 3A may also reveal service needs.

- Find out what occupational health services exist for primary care staff in your locality, and if staff know how to access occupational health services or refer others to them.
- Assess the content and application of your practice's health and safety policy especially the items that relate to staff health. How easy was it to find your policy? When was it last reviewed or amended? Compare the content against a best practice checklist, for example, look at *Occupational Health Matters in General Practice*.[34]

Stage 4: Make and carry out a learning and action plan

- Discuss the updated practice health and safety policy with the local PCO with an occupational health consultant and the practice team. Make final revisions and detailed additions about the health and wellbeing of staff.
- Book dedicated time for discussion with the practice manager about employers' responsibilities in respect of the ill-health of staff and their rehabilitation.
- Read up about patient safety in the National Patient Safety Agency's literature.[35]

Stage 5: Document your learning, competence, performance and standards of service delivery

- Include the revised practice policy for health and safety and wellbeing of staff.
- Make a poster of the practice 'charter' about patient safety for the wall of the staff room.
- Include factual and contemporaneous notes about staff giving concern (anonymised for your PREP/CPD portfolio), the discussions, and the agreed action by the employer (you or the practice manager) and the staff member with follow-up records.

Case study 4.4 continued

Soon after you start to discuss the mistakes that Mrs Burden has made with prescribing, it becomes obvious to you that she has health problems that may be linked to her performance at work. You therefore halt the discussion and advise Mrs Burden to consult her own GP. She makes an appointment the next day and experiences a great relief at being able to unburden herself and not keep up her 'front'. Her GP signs her off sick for two weeks and offers her treatment for her depression. Two months later, she returns to work after receiving the okay from the trust's occupational health department, a much happier person and a more effective nurse.

References

1   World Health Organization (2000) *WHO Guide to Mental Health in Primary Care.* Royal Society of Medicine Press Ltd, London.

2   Goldberg DP and Huxley P (1980) *Mental Illness in the Community: the pathways to psychiatric care.* Tavistock Publications, London.

3   Peveler R, George C, Kinmouth A *et al.* (1999) Effect of anti-depressant drug counselling and information leaflets on adherence to drug treatment in primary care: randomised controlled trial. *British Medical Journal.* **319**: 612–15.

4   Simon G, von Korff M and Barlow W (1995) Health care costs of primary care patients with recognised depression. *Archives of General Psychiatry.* **52**: 850–6.

5   Carney RM, Rich MW, Freedland KE *et al.* (1988) Major depressive disorder predicts cardiac events in patients with coronary artery disease. *Psychosomatic Medicine.* **50**: 627–33.

6   Kessler D, Bennewith O, Lewis G *et al.* (2002) Detection of depression and anxiety in primary care: follow up study. *British Medical Journal.* **325**: 1016–17.

7   Barrett J, Oxman T and Gerber P (1988) The prevalence of psychiatric disorders in primary care practice. *Archives of General Practice.* **45**: 1100–6.

8   Bridges KW and Goldberg DP (1985) Somatic presentation of DSM III psychiatric disorders in primary care. *Journal of Psychosomatic Research.* **29**: 563–9.

9   Chambers R, Boath E and Wakley G (2001) *Mental Health Matters in Primary Care.* Radcliffe Medical Press, Oxford.

10 Katon W, von Korff M, Lin E *et al.* (1992) A randomised trial of psychiatric consultation with distressed high utilisers. *General Hospital Psychiatry.* **14**: 86–98.

11 Dowrick C, Bellon J and Gomez M (2000) GP frequent attendance in Liverpool and Granada: the impact of depressive symptoms. *British Journal of General Practice.* **50**: 361–5.

12 Freemantle N, Long A, Mason J *et al.* (1993) The treatment of depression in primary care. *Effective Health Care Bulletin.* **5**, University of Leeds, Leeds.

13 Tovey D (ed.) (2003) *Clinical Evidence Concise.* Issue 13. BMJ Publishing Group, London.

14 Collier J (2000) The management of postnatal depression. *Drug and Therapeutics Bulletin.* **38(5)**: 33–7.

15 National Institute for Clinical Excellence (NICE) (2004) *Depression: management of depression in primary and secondary care.* NICE, London.

16 National Health Service Executive (2000) *National Service Framework for Mental Health.* Department of Health, London.

17 House A, Owens D and Patchett L (1998) Deliberate self-harm. *Effective Health Care Bulletin.* **4(6)**, University of York, York.

18 Anderson IM, Nutt DJ and Deakin JFW (2000) Evidence based guidelines for treating depressive disorders with antidepressants: a revision of the 1983 British Association for Psychopharmacology guidelines. *Journal of Psychopharmacology.* **14**: 3–20, in: *Guidelines in Practice.* **21**: 151–4.

19 Cornwall P and Scott J (2000) Which clinical practice guidelines for depression? An overview for busy practitioners. *British Journal of General Practice.* **50**: 908–11.

20 MacGillivray S, Arroll B, Hatcher S *et al.* (2003) Efficacy and tolerability of selective serotonin reuptake inhibitors compared with tricyclic antidepressants in depression treated in primary care: systematic review and meta-analysis. *British Medical Journal.* **326**: 1014–17.

21 Lepine JP, Gastpar M, Mendlewicz J *et al.* (1997) Depression in the community: the first pan-European study DEPRES (Depression Research in European Society). *International Clinical Psychopharmacology.* **12(1)**: 19–29.

22 Johnston D (1981) Depression: treatment compliance in general practice. *Acta Psychiatrica Scandinavica.* **Suppl. 63**: 447–53.

23 Marinker M (ed.) (1997) *From Compliance to Concordance: achieving shared goals in medicine taking.* Royal Pharmaceutical Society; Merck, Sharp, and Dohme, London.

24 Wilkinson G, Moore B and Moore P (2000) *Treating People with Depression*. Radcliffe Medical Press, Oxford.

25 National Institute for Clinical Excellence (2003) Guidance on the use of electroconvulsive therapy. *Technology Appraisal* **59**, National Institute for Clinical Excellence, London.

26 Rogers CR (1961) *On Becoming a Person*. Houghton Mifflin, Boston.

27 Ernst E (ed.) (2001) *Complementary and Alternative Medicine – a desktop reference*. Harcourt Health Sciences, London.

28 www.prodigy.nhs.uk/guidance.asp?gt=Depression (accessed 27 April 2005)

29 Collier J (ed.) (2003) Mild depression in general practice: time for a rethink? *Drugs and Therapeutics Bulletin*. **41(8)**: 60–4.

30 Armstrong E (1997) *Primary Mental Health Care Toolkit*. Royal College of General Practitioners Unit for Mental Health Education in Primary Care, London.

31 NHS Centre for Reviews and Dissemination (2002) Improving the recognition and management of depression in primary care. *Effective Health Care Bulletin*, University of York, York.

32 General Practitioners Committee/The NHS Confederation (2003) *New GMS Contract. Investing in general practice*. General Practitioners Committee/NHS Confederation, London.

33 Briddon J (2004) Depression in young women: are you equipped to treat it? *Nursing in Practice*. **17**: 56–8.

34 Chambers R, Moore S, Parker G and Slovak A (2001) *Occupational Health Matters in General Practice*. Radcliffe Medical Press, Oxford.

35 www.npsa.nhs.uk (accessed 27 April 2005)

5

Dementia

Nurses frequently take a lead role in the management of chronic diseases and long-term conditions. Please reread the introduction to Chapter 4 about your need to be qualified for a specialist role or that of a community matron.

Prevalence of dementia

The prevalence of dementia is difficult to establish. In a Canadian study, the rates varied from 3.1% to 29% of the population studied, depending of which of six systems of diagnosis were used.[1] Pooled data from many studies give the prevalence as shown in Table 5.1.

Table 5.1: Prevalence of dementia in the population in Canada

Age group (years)	Prevalence of dementia (cases per 100 people)
65–69	1.4
70–74	2.8
75–79	5.6
80–84	11.1
85+	23.6

That is, about one in every five people over the age of 80 years suffers from dementia. Most studies show no sex difference in prevalence although some show a slightly higher rate of Alzheimer's disease in women. Regional differences appear in many studies but because of the difficulties of precise classification they give a confusing picture. It is suggested that dementia may be less common in rural than in urban areas, and some types of dementia may be more common in some countries.

Case study 5.1

Mrs Grey comes to see you as the health visitor attached to the practice who focuses on the elderly. She tells you that she has been increasingly concerned about her husband's mental state. Since he backed the car into the side of the garage, she has been trying to persuade him to stop driving. She has been asking her daughter to pick them up to go shopping, but this involves both her

---

and her daughter in collusion over the reason, or Mr Grey loses his temper and starts shouting. Then last week, a light bulb went in the hall and Mr Grey, who used to do lots of his own repairs around the house, did not seem to know how to change it. When she tried to tell him to leave it, he became quite aggressive and threw the screwdriver he was holding at her. Later he could not understand why she had been crying and said she was exaggerating, the screwdriver must have slipped out of his hand. He has stopped going out every morning to fetch the paper and then making a cup of tea for them both. She gets quite emotional as she tells you how she misses him reading bits of the paper out to her while they drink their tea, although it always used to annoy her!

What issues you should cover

Take Mrs Grey's concerns seriously, even if you think there may be a possibility of marital discord and exaggeration. It helps to have an account from a relative or other informant if you suspect dementia. As dementia progresses, the patient's own awareness and ability to give a clear history diminishes.

Types of dementia

Many people, including some health professionals, lump all mental decline into a broad category of 'dementia' and look no further. It is important to be as precise as possible, both to identify any reversible causes and to make plans for the future.

Dementia can be divided into two main categories. Those conditions where the dementia is reversible include dehydration, vitamin B deficiency due to poor nutrition or secondary to alcohol abuse, hypothyroidism and head injury. Delirium in acute illness, after surgery, or associated with sleep deprivation can be confused with dementia, but tends to be of shorter duration and relieved by correction of the precipitating event. Severe depression can sometimes mimic dementia.

Irreversible or progressive conditions include those described in Box 5.1.

Box 5.1:   Irreversible or progressive forms of dementia

- *Alzheimer's disease* (AD): the causes of the brain damage of AD are not yet clear but it is known that abnormal amyloid is laid down in the central nervous system. Most people with rare early onset AD have genetic mutations and it is more common in people with Down's syndrome. Symptoms of AD begin slowly with memory problems and become steadily worse. Over time, the brain damage in AD leads to serious problems in thinking, judgement, and ability to carry out daily activities. Speech and personality are also affected. Impairment of cognitive function is commonly accompanied, and occasionally preceded, by deterioration in emotional control, social behaviour or motivation.[2]

- *Lewy body dementia* (LBD): this type of dementia is the possibly second most common cause of dementia in older adults. Lewy bodies are abnormal structures found in certain areas of the brain. This type of dementia can be difficult to diagnose. LBD is characterised by distinct cognitive impairment with fluctuating confusion, disturbance of consciousness, visual hallucinations, delusion, falls and significant parkinsonism. The symptoms tend to come and go, and relatives or professionals may think the individual is pretending to be confused. The condition may be confused with Parkinson's disease because of the symptoms and signs of lack of expression and sensitivity to neuroleptic medication.
- *Multi-infarct or vascular dementia* (MID): in MID, small strokes occur, and blood clots in the blood vessels in the brain cause the death of brain tissue. Symptoms that begin suddenly may be a sign of this kind of dementia. Patients usually have other signs of cardiovascular disease.

The most common form is Alzheimer's disease with about 50–55% of sufferers receiving this diagnosis.[1] About 15–20% have Lewy body or vascular dementia.

There remain around 10% of people with dementia arising from other conditions – about 5% for fronto-temporal dementia including Pick's disease and another 5% for other dementias including acquired immunodeficiency syndrome (AIDS).

- Pick's disease affects the front of the brain, leading to loss of judgement and loss of inhibitions.
- Dementia occurs in the majority of cases of Huntington's disease. This is a hereditary brain disorder causing the loss of cells in the basal ganglia. This cell damage affects cognitive ability (thinking, judgement, memory), movement and emotional control. The symptoms appear gradually, usually in midlife, between the ages of 30 and 50 years.
- Some people with AIDS develop dementia in the later stages of the illness. The AIDS virus itself may attack certain brain cells, and people with AIDS may develop viral infections of the brain because of their weakened immune system.
- The symptoms of Creutzfeldt–Jakob disease (CJD) are similar to those of Alzheimer's disease. An electroencephalogram (EEG) and analysis of the cerebrospinal fluid distinguishes the two conditions.

Clinical priorities

You could invite Mr Grey for a 'well-man' check to assess his physical and mental state. In the early stages of dementia, people may deny that anything is wrong, but sometimes are glad of an opportunity to discuss their fears. In the later stages, people are usually unaware that they have any disability.

Discuss with Mrs Grey whether she feels able to talk to her husband about her concerns about his health. If she can put it in general terms, she may be able to encourage him to attend. However, if Mr Grey has delusions and/or hallucinations, he may have paranoid ideas and be more difficult to help. A history of impairment of function is more likely to imply dementia than just loss of memory.

Identifying and diagnosing dementia[3,4]

It is important not to assume that cognitive impairment equals dementia. A small proportion of people with dementia have an underlying abnormality, such as a brain tumour, that when treated improves cognitive function. Sometimes depression and dementia are confused, particularly in people who become withdrawn and inactive. Depression is common in the early stages of dementia and mental function may improve with treatment of the depression.

Take a history from both the patient and someone who has known the patient for some time. You have the opportunity to hear Mrs Grey's account without Mr Grey being present. This can be important if the patient has delusions, paranoia, denial or is unaware of his dysfunction.

Common causes of cognitive worsening in elderly people are:[5]

- urinary tract, chest, skin or ear infections
- onset or exacerbation of cardiac failure
- drugs, especially prescribed psychiatric or antiparkinsonian drugs and alcohol
- cerebrovascular ischaemia or hypoxia.

Alcohol excess is common in elderly people, especially when they are lonely or lacking in purpose, and other drug use should be considered in some cultures and environments.

Less common causes include:

- severe depression mimicking dementia
- severe anaemia, vitamin B_{12} or folate deficiency
- hypothyroidism
- slow-growing cerebral tumour
- renal failure
- communicating hydrocephalus.

Investigations may include:

- full blood count
- erythrocyte sedimentation rate
- urea and electrolytes
- liver function tests (including gamma-glutamyl transferase)
- vitamin B_{12} and folate, if the mean corpuscular volume is raised
- thyroid function test
- midstream urine
- vision and hearing (may contribute to apparent cognitive impairment)
- ECG
- chest x-ray where indicated to exclude pneumonia or possible chest disease
- CT scan: if symptoms are atypical, there is a recent head injury, clinical suspicion of an underlying tumour, new onset of fits, unexplained focal neurological signs or if antidementia drugs are being considered.

Mental state screening instruments

Tests that are widely used to assess cognitive impairment are the mini-mental state examination (MMSE)[3] or the abbreviated mental test score version,[6] and the six-item cognitive impairment test (6CIT).[7,8] A clock drawing test is becoming increasingly popular and is usually used with the MMSE.[9] Drawing a clock face can reveal deficits in parietal lobe function.

The MMSE consists of 30 questions covering four sections which include: orientation to day, spelling WORLD backwards, recalling three words, and writing a sentence.[3] All other factors should be taken into consideration when interpreting the result, such as a person's background, culture, education and social class, and information from their carers about how they are functioning. Although the MMSE has its limitations, it represents a brief, standardised method by which to grade cognitive mental status. It assesses orientation, attention, immediate and short-term recall, language, and the ability to follow simple verbal and written commands. Scoring allows the individual to be rated as to cognitive function, and the results of successive tests to be compared over time.

The abbreviated mental test score (AMT) is a quick way to evaluate cognitive function in general practice to screen for dementia or monitor its progression.[4] The AMT consists of a set of 10 questions for the patient and takes about 10 minutes to administer and complete (*see* Box 5.2). A cognitively intact person should answer the 10 questions correctly, whereas a score below 6 indicates likely cognitive impairment.

Box 5.2:   The abbreviated mental test score[4]

Each correct answer scores one point

  1 Age
  2 Time to nearest hour
  3 An address to be repeated by the patient at the end of the test
  4 Year
  5 Name of hospital or residence etc where patient is situated
  6 Recognition of two persons e.g. doctor, home help, etc
  7 Date of birth
  8 Year that the First World War started
  9 Name of present monarch
10 Count backwards from 20 to 1

The 6CIT consists of six questions that are simple and non-cultural and do not require any complex interpretation (*see* Box 5.3). GPs have found that the 6CIT is more appropriate for those with mild dementia than the MMSE.[5] The 6CIT can be loaded on the practice computer as a Windows-based program.[10]

Box 5.3: The 6CIT test

Try to perform the test in a quiet place with no obvious clock or calendar visible to the patient. Score the test as in the list below.

- Ask question 1 and then question 2 (*see* below).
- Tell the patient you are going to tell them a fictional address which you would like them to try to memorise and then repeat back to you afterwards. Say the address. Make sure the patient is able to repeat the address correctly before moving on and warn them to try to memorise it as you are going to ask them to repeat it again in a few minutes. No score is made at this stage.
- Ask the patient the time; if they get within 60 minutes of the correct time then they score 0, if not then score 3.
- Ask the patient to count backwards from 20 to 1. If they do this correctly score 0. If they make one error score 2; two or more errors score 4.
- Ask the patient to say the months of the year backwards starting with December. Give them plenty of time for this and it doesn't matter if they keep saying the months forward in order to get the answer.
- Finally ask them to repeat the address back to you. The address is broken into five fragments and is scored for each error (*see* list below).

1 What year is it?
   Correct 0; incorrect 4
2 What month is it?
   Correct 0; incorrect 3
3 Remember the following address: John Brown, 42 West Street, Bedford
4 What time is it?
   Correct 0; incorrect 3
5 Count backwards from 20 to 1
   Correct 0; one error 2; more than one error 4
6 Say the months of the year backwards
   Correct 0; one error 2; more than one error 4
7 Repeat memory phrase
   Correct 0; one error 2; two errors 4; three errors 6; four errors 8; all incorrect 10

Interpreting the score
0–7: normal
8–9: mild cognitive impairment – refer to memory clinic
10–28: significant cognitive impairment

The Clifton Assessment Procedures for the Elderly (CAPE) are useful to give a profile for a patient but do not provide a score.[11,12] It is quick and easy to fill in together with observations from carers (*see* Box 5.4). It can be used to estimate the likelihood of strain on the carer. It is important to regularly review the patient's ability to perform daily tasks safely, behavioural problems and general physical condition.

Box 5.4: The Clifton Assessment Procedures for the Elderly (CAPE)[11,12]

Information/orientation

- Can you give me your name?
- Can you tell the name of where you are now?
- Who is the prime minister now?
- What day is it?
- Can you give me your address?
- Can you tell the address of where you are now?
- Who is the president of the United States?
- What month is it?
- Can you tell me your date of birth?
- Can you tell the name of the town/city where you are now?
- What colour is the flag?
- What year is it?

Physical disability

- When bathing or dressing, he/she requires:
  - no help
  - some help
  - maximum help
- With regard to walking, he/she:
  - shows no signs of weakness
  - walks slowly without aid, or uses a stick
  - is unable to walk (or if able to walk needs a frame, crutches or someone by their side)
- He/she is incontinent of urine and/or faeces (day or night):
  - never
  - sometimes (once or twice a week)
  - frequently (three times a week or more)
- He/she is in bed during the day (bed does not include couch, settee etc):
  - never
  - sometimes
  - almost always
- He/she is confused (unable to find way around, loses possessions etc):
  - almost never
  - sometimes
  - almost always
- Left to his/her own devices, his/her appearance (clothes and/or hair) is:
  - almost never disorderly
  - sometimes disorderly
  - almost always disorderly

Some areas have memory clinics – of which some see only patients at an early stage of dementia, and others perform multidisciplinary assessments at any stage of dementia. You should know if there is a clinic near you and what the criteria are for referral.[11]

The importance of early diagnosis[13]

Early diagnosis allows the patient and family to plan for the future and identify outside sources of assistance. As potentially useful and proven treatments become available, early diagnosis of dementia will become increasingly important. Although screening all elderly patients for dementia is not warranted, being alert for cognitive and functional decline is a prudent way of recognising dementia in its early stage. Knowing the diagnosis provides carers with an explanation for their relative's behaviour and stops them from blaming themselves or the relative.

In addition, early detection may lead to the detection and treatment of co-existing medical conditions that can be mistaken for dementia or that may be contributing to its severity.

The primary care team has a central role in the diagnosis and ongoing care of dementia. Its roles in diagnosis and management include:

- identifying people who have suspected dementia
- excluding treatable causes
- referring to specialist psychiatric services when the diagnosis is uncertain
- providing information about the diagnosis and prognosis of dementia
- assessing the informal carer's ability to cope
- providing information about available services and benefits
- helping with access to, and co-ordination of, a range of support services
- providing emotional support to informal carers
- treating co-existing conditions as they occur
- monitoring and co-ordinating care of the individual with dementia
- prescribing new drugs for dementia in association with the physician initiating treatment.

Consider referral to social services for practical help, needs assessment, formal care planning, home help and day care and help with respite, placement and benefits.

Classification of dementia[14]

Dementia is classified as minimal, mild, moderate or severe dementia. Each stage merges into the next one. Dementia may be temporarily worse with intercurrent illness.

Minimal dementia

A person with 'minimal' dementia has some difficulty in recalling recent events and may be prone to mislaying or losing things. A person with minimal dementia is usually still independent and care is probably not needed.

Mild dementia

A person with 'mild' dementia has most or all of the following signs and symptoms:

- difficulty in recalling recent information
- limited or patchy disorientation in time and place
- impaired problem solving, reasoning and the ability to manage everyday activities.

In the later stages of mild dementia, some degree of care will usually be required.

Moderate dementia

A person with 'moderate' dementia has most of the following signs and symptoms:

- severely impaired reasoning, problem solving and recall of recent events
- disorientated in time and place
- speech slightly unclear, but not to a marked degree
- not able to manage housework, shopping and finances independently
- needs help with dressing and other self-care
- may be occasionally incontinent.

Daily care is usually required for those with moderate dementia.

Severe dementia

A person with 'severe' dementia:

- is totally disorientated
- is incapable of recall, reasoning and self-care
- is unable to communicate in normal speech
- may fail to recognise close relatives
- is almost invariably incontinent, apathetic and inert.

The person with severe dementia may become immobile, and will be totally incapable of being independent. Continual care and supervision are usually required.

The need for care depends on how long an individual can remain living alone or being independent. Regularly assess risk, balancing safety and independence. Discuss planning of legal and financial affairs. Attendance Allowance can usually be claimed. An information sheet is available from the Alzheimer's Society.[11] The needs of an individual tend to vary from time to time, as there may be episodes of severely disturbed behaviour. Health and social care services need to be flexible.

Case study 5.1 continued

Mrs Grey telephones you to say that Mr Grey has agreed to attend for a 'well-man' check with the practice nurse. You brief the practice nurse who has been trained in administering the 6CIT loaded on the computer. She arranges for Mr Grey to have some screening blood and urine tests and to attend the GP for the results following his 'well-man' check. The results suggest that he has mild dementia, with some awareness of his decline in ability, and is depressed.

Mr Grey agrees to be referred to the memory clinic, as there might be a possibility of receiving treatment initiated by the specialist. In the meantime, he agrees to try an antidepressant and to see the GP again about this in a couple of weeks. You suggest Mrs Grey contacts Age Concern[15] or the Alzheimer's Society[11] so that she can start making some longer-term plans.

Treatment of dementia

The North of England evidence-based guidelines development project and the Scottish Intercollegiate Guidelines Network (SIGN) give similar recommendations for pharmacological treatments.[16,17] Neuroleptic drugs are the mainstay of pharmacological treatment for Alzheimer's disease but they do have side-effects such as parkinsonism, drowsiness, tardive dyskinesia, falls accelerating cognitive decline, and severe neuroleptic sensitivity reactions. Patients with dementia from Lewy bodies are more sensitive to the side-effects of neuroleptic medication and should not be prescribed these medications, so an accurate diagnosis is imperative.[16] Behavioural problems (e.g. aggression or restlessness) change with the course of the dementia, therefore medication should be reviewed regularly to see if it is still needed.[18]

The current National Institute for Clinical Excellence (NICE) recommendations about donepezil, rivastigmine and galantamine in the treatment of Alzheimer's disease (*see* Box 5.5)[19] are due to be reappraised in 2005 and there appears to be some dispute about whether the small advantages of medication are cost-effective.

Box 5.5:   NICE recommendations for treatment with donepezil, rivastigmine and galantamine in Alzheimer's disease[19]

1   Diagnosis that the form of dementia is AD must be made in a specialist clinic according to standard diagnostic criteria.
2   Assessment in a specialist clinic, including tests of cognitive, global and behavioural functioning and of activities of daily living, should be made before the drug is prescribed.
3   Clinicians should exercise judgement about the likelihood of compliance; in general, a carer or care-worker who is in sufficient contact with the patient to ensure compliance should be a minimum requirement.
4   Only specialists (including old age psychiatrists, neurologists, and care of the elderly physicians) should initiate treatment.
5   Carers' views of the patient's condition at baseline and follow up should be sought. If GPs are to take over prescribing, it is recommended that they should do so under an agreed shared-care protocol with clear treatment endpoints.
6   A further assessment should be made, usually two to four months after reaching a maintenance dose of the drug. Following this assessment the drug should be continued only where there has been an improvement or no deterioration in MMSE score, together with evidence of global improvement on the basis of behavioural and/or functional assessment.

7   Patients who continue on the drug should be reviewed by MMSE score and global, functional and behavioural assessment every six months. The drug should normally only be continued while their MMSE score remains above 12 points, and their global, functional and behavioural condition remains at a level where the drug is considered to be having a worthwhile effect. When the MMSE score falls below 12 points, patients should not normally be prescribed any of these drugs. Any review involving MMSE assessment should be undertaken by an appropriate specialist team, unless there are locally agreed protocols for shared care.

Treatment with olanzapine, risperidone or carbamazepine has been tried if agitation, delusions or hallucinations are present.[2] The adverse effects of atypical antipsychotic drugs, particularly in increasing the tendency to fall and the incidence of diabetes means that non-pharmaceutical measures should be tried first. Moreover, recent evidence about the increased risk of mortality and stroke in people treated with olanzapine has prompted a change in recommendations. Olanzapine is now not approved for the treatment of dementia-related psychosis.[20]

Low-dose aspirin (75–150 mg daily) may be indicated in MID.

Mr and Mrs Grey will want to discuss what they can do themselves while awaiting the decision at the memory clinic. *Clinical Evidence* evaluates the following treatments as beneficial.[2]

• An extract of ginkgo biloba, taken as a 40 mg tablet three times daily before food, seems to be effective for people with dementia and is well tolerated. The 'number needed to treat' (NNT) calculation predicts that about seven patients with dementia have to be treated with 120 mg of ginkgo extract daily for one year for one of them to have an improvement which they would not have had with placebo treatment. That level of improvement is equivalent to a six-month delay in the progression of the dementia.[21]

• There seems to be an association between high levels of serum homocysteine and low levels of serum folate and dementia. The conclusion of one review was that taking a daily multivitamin is likely to prevent cardiovascular disease, cancer and possibly dementia.[22]

• Reality orientation presents the patient with orientation information through techniques such as the use of calendars, cueing, and reinforcement by repetition of information, and is thought to provide the patient with a greater understanding of his or her environment (*see* Box 5.6).

Box 5.6:   Reality orientation
• Surround people with Alzheimer's disease with familiar objects that can be used to stimulate their memory. Other materials, such as a family scrapbook, flash cards, Scrabble games, a globe, large-piece jigsaw puzzles, and illustrated, large-print dictionaries, also help.

- Another tool, the reality-orientation board, is any board with a surface on which information can be changed easily, such as a blackboard, a pegboard, or an erasable memo board. Both the caregiver and the person with Alzheimer's disease fill in information such as current day of the week, date, and year, and the weather.
- For persons who are severely confused, the focus is on less complicated information, such as their own name and address, the name of their caregiver, colours, and identification of everyday objects.
- Reality orientation is around-the-clock therapy; the caregiver and anyone should be encouraged to apply the techniques. General guidelines include the following:
  - treat people with memory impairment with respect. Do not talk down to them or treat them like children
  - every conversation you have with the person should include mention of the time, day of the week, and names of familiar people and objects.

People with Alzheimer's should be encouraged to perform activities of daily living, that is, getting dressed, eating and taking care of personal hygiene, and should be complimented on all such attempts.

Other forms of therapy have unknown effectiveness and are still under review. Reminiscence work and music therapy are unlikely to harm and may make Mrs Grey and her family feel that they are contributing to Mr Grey's care in a positive way. The Alzheimer's Society will be able to keep Mrs Grey up to date on the latest information.[11]

Collecting data to demonstrate your learning, competence, performance and standards of service delivery

Example cycle of evidence 5.1

- Focus: relationships with patients
- Other relevant foci: maintaining good nursing practice; working with colleagues; probity

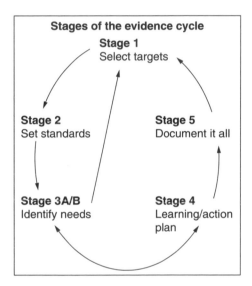

Stages of the evidence cycle

Stage 1
Select targets

Stage 2
Set standards

Stage 5
Document it all

Stage 3A/B
Identify needs

Stage 4
Learning/action plan

Case study 5.2

The triage nurse has referred Mr French to you, the district nurse, as he is already known to you and on your caseload for Zoladex injections and dressings. You are aware he is on medication for prostate problems, varicose ulcers and osteoarthritis. She tells you that usually Mr French, who has Alzheimer's disease, rings demanding visits for various ailments that he has forgotten are all being treated. Usually when someone rings back, Mrs French says wearily that he has no new problems and not to bother. Mrs French does much valuable work with the local branch of the Alzheimer's Society and has mobilised all possible assistance for her husband. This time when you ring, she explains that her brother-in-law is visiting from France and is insisting on a visit, as he believes she and the practice have been ignoring his requests for help.

When you attend, the brother-in-law and Mr French are quite intimidating. The brother-in-law tells you that he was not aware of his brother's deteriorating function. He wants the four-layer bandages redone so that he can see what is wrong with his brother's legs and tells you that he has written down a list of drugs that are, as he puts it, 'essential'. The list includes galantamine, ginkgo biloba, folic acid and trazodone. You try to explain that Mr French had been on donepezil, but had shown no improvement, so it had been stopped. The brother-in-law brushes aside your explanations as 'money-saving'. You find yourself uncomfortably agreeing to ask the GP to review him. You can see Mrs French behind the two of them, shaking her head at you.

> This is just an example. Keep your task simple. You could choose three or four cycles of evidence to demonstrate your competence each year.

Stage 1: Select your aspirations for good practice

The excellent nurse:

- seeks consent before sharing information
- provides or arranges investigations or treatment when necessary
- refers to another practitioner when indicated
- keeps open lines of communication with colleagues
- works with colleagues to monitor and maintain the quality of care provided
- makes sure that others understand his or her professional status and speciality, what roles and responsibilities he/she has and who is responsible for each aspect of the patient's care.

Stage 2: Set the standards for your outcomes

Outcomes might include:

- the way learning is applied
- a learnt skill
- a protocol
- a strategy that is implemented
- meeting recommended standards.

- Demonstrate consistent best practice in the management of patients with dementia.
- Document best practice in managing the concerns of relatives and seeking consent for the sharing of information.

Stage 3A: Identify your learning needs

- Self-assess your knowledge about the management of patients with dementia.
- Keep a reflective diary about how you handled your irritation over the relative's assumption that you, the practice and Mrs French were providing inadequate care.
- Think how best to obtain consent to disclosure of medical information when a patient is accompanied by a relative and has cognitive deficiencies.

Stage 3B: Identify your service needs

Any of the needs assessment exercises in 3A may also reveal service needs.

- Look at the practice guidelines for review of patients with dementia.
- Discuss with the practice team whether your visit to Mr French was appropriate under the circumstances.

Stage 4: Make and carry out a learning and action plan

- Read up on the current NICE guidelines[19] and the evidence in *Clinical Evidence Concise*.[2]
- Arrange a tutorial with the care of the elderly mental health team.
- Discuss the practice guidelines for review of patients with dementia at a practice meeting.
- Attend workshops on best practice on consent to disclosure of medical information and managing the concerns of relatives.

Stage 5: Document your learning, competence, performance and standards of service delivery

- Keep a copy of the practice guidelines for review of patients with dementia.
- Include notes from your reflective diary on how you handled your irritation over the relatives' comments.
- Keep your notes from the workshops on best practice on consent to disclosure of medical information and managing the concerns of relatives.
- Keep notes from the tutorial with the care of the elderly mental health team.

Case study 5.2 continued

You ask one of the receptionists, who lives near Mrs French, to drop round a copy of the patient information from the NICE recommendations,[19] together with a printout of the latest information from *Clinical Evidence Concise*[2] for her brother-in-law to read that evening.

The following day, you discuss Mr French's management with the GP, who points out that Mr French had had an extended appointment to review all his ailments in the surgery only two months previously. The GP thinks that a family conference with the sons and daughter who live nearer and visit more often may be required to prevent interference from a relative who has not seen his brother-in-law for several years. He will discuss this with Mrs French.

The procedure for review of patients with dementia by the practice team is found to be working well and does not require any change.

Following the workshops on managing the concerns of relatives and obtaining consent from patients with cognitive impairment, you feel more confident that you will manage this type of consultation better in future.

Example cycle of evidence 5.2

- Focus: clinical care
- Other relevant foci: relationships with carers; relationships with patients

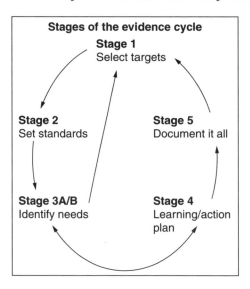

Stages of the evidence cycle

Stage 1
Select targets

Stage 2
Set standards

Stage 5
Document it all

Stage 3A/B
Identify needs

Stage 4
Learning/action plan

Case study 5.3

The GP has referred Gladys Pad to you as the district nurse for a continence assessment. When you arrive, her husband greets you at the front door looking frazzled. You notice an odour of urine as you enter the home, and the house appears untidy with dishes in the kitchen sink. Mr Pad apologises for the mess but he tells you he has 'little time for chores as I have to keep an eye on Gladys all the time these days'.

This is just an example. Keep your task simple. You could choose three or four cycles of evidence to demonstrate your competence each year.

Stage 1: Select your aspirations for good practice

The excellent nurse:

- monitors and co-ordinates care of individuals with dementia
- makes appropriate and timely referrals
- considers ways to reduce stress on those caring for patients.

Stage 2: Set the standards for your outcomes

Outcomes might include:

- the way learning is applied
- a learnt skill
- a protocol
- a strategy that is implemented
- meeting recommended standards.

- Carers' needs are always assessed and documented.
- All members of the practice team are aware of support and advice available to carers of patients with dementia.

Stage 3A: Identify your learning needs

- Self-assess your knowledge of the support available for patients with dementia and for their carers in your locality.
- Audit 10 consecutive patients' notes for documented assessment of carer needs.
- Gain feedback from colleagues and/or team members on the quality of your assessments of carer needs.

Stage 3B: Identify your service needs

Any of the needs assessment exercises in 3A may also reveal service needs.

- Establish what advice other practice team members give to carers of patients with dementia by asking carers for feedback on advice received and the perceived usefulness of the advice.
- Monitor the availability and accessibility of day care programmes in your area by reviewing waiting times to access a place on a day care programme.

Stage 4: Make and carry out a learning and action plan

- Gather information on support for carers from the community mental health team, social services and voluntary agencies, and give a presentation of this information at a practice meeting.
- Audit the time from referral to a day care programme to the date a patient commences on the programme.
- Discuss with the primary care organisation (PCO) the results of your review of day care provision in the area.

Stage 5: Document your learning, competence, performance and standards of service delivery

- Document the results of audit of time from referral to commencement of day care.
- Keep the results of the audit of patient notes for documented assessment of carers.
- Keep a record of feedback from colleagues on the quality of your assessments of carer needs.
- Make notes on discussions with the PCO on day care provision in the area.
- Keep a copy of your presentation to the practice team of information to support carers.

Case study 5.3 continued

You complete the continence assessment and discuss with Mr Pad what support is available to him. With his agreement you refer them to social services for day care and home help, and you give Mr Pad the contacts for the Alzheimer support group in your area. The PCO thanks you for highlighting the issues with day care provision, and plans to include it in its commissioning process.

Example cycle of evidence 5.3

*   Focus: teaching and training
*   Other relevant foci: relationships with patients and carers; maintaining good nursing practice

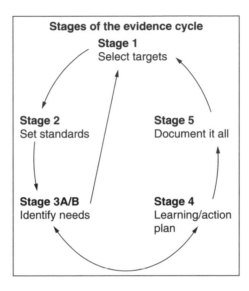

Case study 5.4

A nursing student is sitting in your surgery when Miss Wisp arrives with her neighbour Mrs Worthy. Miss Wisp says that she just gets anxious, and is just a bit forgetful nowadays. Mrs Worthy takes over and explains that she pops in to keep an eye on her 68-year-old neighbour. Miss Wisp seems fine one day but 'totally with the fairies' on another day. She reminds Miss Wisp of various episodes recently – putting on her clothes over her nightie, burning out a saucepan that she put empty onto the cooking ring, spending hours looking for her keys or her glasses that she thinks have been hidden by someone who has come into the house, forgetting to pay bills and not eating properly. Miss Wisp breaks down in tears and says she doesn't understand why she cannot cope some days. Her niece has stopped coming to see her after she accused Miss Wisp of playing at being helpless to get attention. You explain to the nursing student that you are conducting a memory test. Miss Wisp manages the abbreviated mental test score with only one error. The student says 'I don't think there's much wrong with your memory' and Miss Wisp looks as if she will burst into tears again. You intervene to arrange some investigations and ask to see her again – you suggest she attends on a 'not-good' day to assess her again and Mrs Worthy agrees to bring her again.

This is just an example. Keep your task simple. You could choose three or four cycles of evidence to demonstrate your competence each year.

Stage 1: Select your aspirations for good practice

The excellent nurse:

- helps to educate other colleagues at all levels
- does not undermine the confidence of juniors or students
- treats patients with courtesy and consideration
- keeps his/her knowledge up to date.

Stage 2: Set the standards for your outcomes

Outcomes might include:

- the way learning is applied
- a learnt skill
- a protocol
- a strategy that is implemented
- meeting recommended standards.

- Demonstrate an active involvement in the training of another.
- Behave in a courteous way to patients and students.
- Be up to date with knowledge about dementia.

Stage 3A: Identify your learning needs

- Review your teaching skills by obtaining consent to videotape a tutorial with the nursing student and exchanging videos with another trainer for mutual peer review.
- Check that your knowledge about dementia is correct and up to date by checking against best practice.
- Obtain feedback from the students, anonymised via the higher education institution.
- Check whether you have the skills to guide the student to manage this type of problem.

Stage 3B: Identify your service needs

> Any of the needs assessment exercises in 3A may also reveal service needs.

- Find out what help the health visitor and district nurse can give the nursing student to learn about how patients with dementia can be helped to manage at home, and what options are available if they cannot manage at home.
- Ask the practice manager who supervises the provision of patient literature to review with the nursing student the usefulness of the literature on dementia available in the practice to patients and carers.

Stage 4: Make and carry out a learning and action plan

- Read about dementia, and particularly about the diagnosis of LBD.
- Prepare and give a tutorial for the nursing student on the diagnosis and management of dementia.
- Attend an update course for community practice educators (CPEs) and mentors.
- Read the literature on dementia, selected as most useful by the nursing student and practice nurse, so that you can recommend it appropriately to patients and carers.

Stage 5: Document your learning, competence, performance and standards of service delivery

- Keep a record of the results of the peer review of your tutorial and feedback from students.
- Record your new knowledge about dementia.
- Keep a list of the available selected patient information literature on dementia.
- Keep your notes on the CPEs' and mentors' update course.

Case study 5.4 continued

You give a tutorial to the nursing student with your new knowledge. You learn some more from the work the nursing student has done to find out the literature available to patients with dementia and their carers. The student is amazed at the complexity of the job the practice nurse is expected to do, and acknowledges that she was less than tactful telling Miss Wisp that there was nothing wrong with her memory when she hears about the variable nature of the cognitive changes in LBD.

You have a more appropriate supply of literature for patients with dementia and their carers. You feel that your teaching skills have been improved by the attendance at the course and the reviews and reflections about the task.

References

1   Erikinjuntti T, Østbye T, Steenhuis R *et al.* (1997) The effect of different diagnostic criteria on the prevalence of dementia. *New England Journal of Medicine.* **337**: 1667–74.

2   Tovey D (ed.) (2003) *Clinical Evidence Concise.* Issue 13. BMJ Publishing Group, London. www.clinicalevidence.com (accessed 27 April 2005)

3   Thistlethwaite J (2000) Dementia: the role of the primary care team. *Update.* **17 August**: 150–4.

4   Folstein MF, Folstein SE and McHugh PR (1975) Mini-mental state: a practical method for grading the cognitive state of patients for the clinician. *Journal of Psychiatric Research.* **12**: 189–98.

5   Foord-Kelcey G (ed.) (2004) Diagnosis and management of dementia in primary care. *Guidelines.* **22**: 143–4. www.eguidelines.co.uk

6   Research Unit of the Royal College of Physicians and the British Geriatrics Society (1992) *Standardised Assessment Scales for Elderly People.* The Royal College of Physicians of London and the British Geriatrics Society, London.

7   Brooke P and Bullock R (1999) Validation of the 6 item cognitive impairment test. *International Journal of Geriatric Psychiatry.* **14**: 936–40.

8   Brooke P (2000) A better test for cognitive loss. *The Practitioner.* **244**: 389 and 463.

9   Sunderland T, Hill JL, Mellow AM *et al.* (1989) Clock drawing in Alzheimer's disease. A novel measure of dementia severity. *Journal of the American Geriatric Society.* **37**: 725–9.

10 www.kingshill-research.org/kresearch/6cit.asp (accessed 27 April 2005)

11 Alzheimer's Disease Society www.alzheimers.org.uk (accessed 27 April 2005)

12 www.ehr.chime.ucl.ac.uk/demcare/cape.html (accessed 27 April 2005)

13 Iliffe S, Manthorpe J and Eden A (2003) Sooner or later? Issues in the early diagnosis of dementia in general practice: a qualitative study. *Family Practice.* **20**: 376–81.

14 Audit Commission (2000) *Forget Me Not – mental health services for older people.* Audit Commission, London.

15 www.ageconcern.org.uk (accessed 27 April 2005)

16 Eccles M, Clarke J and Livingston M (1998) North of England evidence based guidelines development project: guideline for the primary care management of dementia. *British Medical Journal.* **317**: 802–8.

17 Scottish Intercollegiate Guidelines Network (1998) *Interventions in the Management of Behavioural and Psychological Aspects of Dementia.* Scottish Intercollegiate Guidelines Network, Edinburgh. www.sign.ac.uk (accessed 27 April 2005)

18 World Health Organization (2000) *WHO Guide to Mental Health in Primary Care.* The Royal Society of Medicine Press Ltd, London.

19 Technology Appraisal Guidance (2003) *Guidance on the Use of Donepezil, Rivastigmine and Galantamine for the Treatment of Alzheimer's Disease.* National Institute for Clinical Excellence, London. www.nice.org.uk (accessed 27 April 2005)

20 www.emea.eu.int/htms/human/drugalert/drugalert.htm (accessed 27 April 2005)

21 Moore A, McQuay H and Muir Gray JA (1998) Dementia diagnosis and treatment. *Bandolier.* **5(2)**: 2–3.

22 Moore A, McQuay H and Muir Gray JA (1999) Folate, homocysteine and dementia. *Bandolier.* **6(9)**: 1–2.

6

Alcohol problems

Nurses frequently take a lead role in the management of chronic diseases and long-term conditions. Please reread the introduction to Chapter 4 about your need to be qualified for a specialist role or that of community matron.

Alcohol misuse is a major public health concern and has a huge impact on the economy, both in relation to healthcare costs and lost productivity at work.[1] Primary care settings are ideally suited to help both identify and treat patients with alcohol misuse problems, having the dual advantage of seeing large numbers of patients and being able to provide them with opportunistic health promotion.[2] On average 360 patients who are misusing alcohol are seen each year in general practice. Research evidence suggests approximately 20% of patients presenting to primary care are likely to be hazardous drinkers.[2]

Case study 6.1

Ms Quaff is a 39-year-old professional woman who consults you, the nurse practitioner, complaining of severe anxiety. You have not seen her before even though she has been registered with the surgery for three years. You find out that she is the human resources director of a large retail firm, travels a great deal and is barely at home for more then three consecutive days. She feels anxious every morning and finds that the symptoms persist throughout the day. She finds it difficult to sleep at night, not helped by her frequent travelling across time zones. She begins to cry, and what emerges is that she may be drinking too much. You ask her more and find out that she consumes on average five 'small' gins most evenings and around a bottle of wine with her meal every evening.

What issues you should cover

Around 4% of the adult population are 'harmful drinkers' causing imminent risk to health. A further 23% are described as 'hazardous' drinkers, at increasing risk of health and injury, a considerable 8.8 million people in England (*see* Box 6.1 for definitions).

Box 6.1:   Definitions of alcohol abuse

- *Hazardous drinking*: consuming 22–50 units a week for men and 15–35 units a week for women, and carries increasing risk to health.
- *Harmful drinking*: consuming more than 50 units a week for men and 35 units a week for women and causing imminent risk to health.
- *Binge drinking*: men regularly drinking 10 or more units in a single session, and women regularly drinking 7 or more units in a single session. This is more than double the daily sensible drinking benchmark.
- *Alcohol dependence* (the term used in preference to 'alcoholism'): periodic or chronic intoxication, uncontrolled craving, tolerance resulting in dose increase and dependence on drinking alcohol.

The term 'hazardous drinking' is widely used and is synonymous with 'at-risk drinking'. Hazardous drinkers are unlikely to seek treatment for their drinking, and usually they do not actually need treatment as such. What they do need is early identification and early intervention, based on proven clinical techniques.

Presentation[3]

Primary care workers should be alerted, by certain presentations and physical signs, to the possibility that alcohol is a contributory factor and should ask about alcohol consumption. You may find it helpful to use a validated screening tool such as AUDIT, which can be incorporated into a general health interview, lifestyle questionnaire or medical history.[3] This and other screening tools are available from the Alcohol Concern website.[4] Patients who abuse alcohol may present in primary care with:

- depressed mood or failed treatment for depression
- nervousness
- insomnia
- physical complications such as stomach ulcer, gastritis, liver disease, hypertension
- accidents or injuries due to alcohol misuse
- poor memory or concentration
- evidence of self-neglect such as poor hygiene
- legal or social problems such as marital problems, domestic violence, child abuse or neglect, absence from work
- signs of withdrawal from alcohol: sweating, tremors, morning sickness, hallucinations, seizures
- a request for help: family members because the patient who is abusing alcohol denies problem, or the person themself presents for help or advice.

History taking

Ms Quaff is obviously drinking a lot of alcohol. It is important to try and determine the extent that her drinking has become a problem, that is, falling into the 'problem drinking' category, and whether and how dependent she is. Complete the alcohol history, obtaining as accurate an account as possible of how much, when and in what circumstances she drinks. So, for example, when she says small gin, is this a home measure, which is often much more than a single pub measure, or is it the small bottle (equivalent to a double measure) often sold or given free in planes? Does she drink a bottle of wine every night in addition to the five gins? If one unit is a single measure of spirit, half a pint of normal strength lager or a small glass of wine (a bottle has about five glasses) then she is drinking between 10 and 15 units per day or 70–105 units per week, well above the recommended level for women (*see* Figure 6.1).

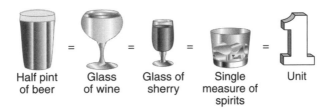

Half pint   Glass   Glass of   Single   Unit
of beer   of wine   sherry   measure of
                                   spirits

Figure 6.1:   Units contained in different drinks.

Try and find out how long Ms Quaff has been following this pattern. Look especially for the following:[3]

- stereotyped drinking pattern (same drink, same time)
- craving
- early morning drinking
- drinking to offset uncomfortable withdrawal symptoms such as 'the shakes'
- loss of control, often associated with blackouts
- tolerance: able to drink large quantities, rapidly developing even after a period of abstinence
- withdrawal symptoms, such as early morning retching, headache, sweating, shakes (these symptoms are often misinterpreted as anxiety).

Complications of alcohol use[5]

The complications of excess alcohol use affect every organ within the body. With Ms Quaff, focus on her psychological issues, such as depression, anxiety and panic attacks. Discuss the possible hazards of hypertension, menstrual disorders, gastritis, etc (*see* Table 6.1). Investigations may reveal abnormal liver function tests.

Investigations

Biological markers of alcohol problems are useful when there is a reason to believe that self-reporting may be inaccurate, and can be useful to motivate patients to review their drinking and to consider change. They can also be used to monitor patients' progress in reducing their drinking.

Table 6.1:   Estimates of proportion of death attributable to alcohol from various conditions in England and Wales[6]

Cause of death	Percentage of deaths attributable to alcohol
Cancer of the oesophagus	14–75
Cancer of the liver	15–29
Cancer of the female breast	3–4
Hypertension	5–11
Chronic pancreatitis	60–84
Acute pancreatitis	24–35
Falls	23–35
Drowning	30–38
Fire injuries	38–45
Suicide	27–41
Assault	27–47

The three most commonly identified, and indeed most frequently used, markers of alcohol misuse are elevation of the erythrocyte mean corpuscular volume (MCV), and increases in serum aspartate aminotransferase (AST) and gamma glutamyl transpeptidase (GGT) levels. A number of other non-specific abnormalities such as hyperuricaemia and hypertriglyceridaemia may also be observed.

Case study 6.1 continued

Ms Quaff has been drinking heavily for seven years and has not had an alcohol-free day during this period. She realises that it is now getting out of hand but hadn't realised what a problem it actually was until she started talking to you. She wants to know what to do, whether to stop completely or to reduce her intake. Physical examination has shown that she is hypertensive. You arrange baseline blood investigations and arrange to see her again. In the meantime you suggest that she keeps an alcohol diary indicating when she drinks and the quantity, and give her some information (*see* Box 6.2) and a leaflet about 'women and alcohol'.[7]

Box 6.2:   Information about women and drinking alcohol

- More than 60% of all sexually transmitted diseases (STDs) and unplanned pregnancies among students result from sexual encounters while one or more of the partners is drinking – interfering with adequate sexual decision making and practice of personal protection.
- More than 75% of 'acquaintance' rape and 60% of 'stranger' rape involve alcohol – either the perpetrator and/or the woman is drinking.

- The majority of domestic violence, including wife battering and child abuse, is associated with alcohol overuse.
- Women are more discreet at hiding their excessive alcohol intake, and hence present for treatment much later than their male counterparts.
- Women are more likely to experience multiple dependence, especially on benzodiazepines and antidepressants.
- Treatment of alcohol abuse in women is more likely to include other co-morbid factors such as anorexia nervosa, depression, and anxiety.

Case study 6.1 continued

Ms Quaff returns two weeks later. Her liver function tests and full blood count are consistent with high alcohol use and her cholesterol is raised at 7.8 mmol/l.

Ms Quaff claims to only drink in the evenings, never to have had a drink in the morning and has not had blackouts or shakes. Her drink diary shows that she indeed does drink around 10 units of alcohol a night, though more if she is on business when it can rise to 20 units.

She has already begun to reduce her alcohol consumption, has talked to her bosses and asked to be transferred to a different section in the organisation, one that doesn't require as much travel. She was very grateful to you for uncovering her high alcohol consumption – something she had been worrying about for some time but was too ashamed to admit. She didn't realise how much damage it was doing to her though.

Giving advice

Ms Quaff is drinking excessively but may not be dependent. You suggest that though her drinking is excessive, controlled drinking may be a realistic option. Tactics include:

- drinking modestly, no more than two standard drinks per day, with one or two alcohol-free days a week
- spacing drinks with non-alcoholic beverages or low-alcohol drinks
- eating before drinking and eating when drinking
- quenching thirst on water or soft drinks
- avoiding joining in with 'rounds'.

Abstinence is recommended if there is established alcohol dependence, marked physical damage, or when controlled drinking has failed.

Brief and minimal interventions[8,9]

You have already started intervening just by taking a history and listening to her worries. Research has shown that spending even a few minutes with a patient, offering advice on reducing consumption and motivating in a non-judgemental fashion, can bring about change.[10] Interventions can be from a few minutes to several half-hour sessions; the term 'minimal brief interventions' is used to describe sessions of up to five minutes provided by a primary care health professional.

A meta-analysis found that excessive drinkers who received brief intervention were twice as likely to moderate their drinking when compared to excessive drinkers who did not receive any intervention.[10] 'Brief intervention' is generally restricted to four or fewer sessions, each session lasting from a few minutes to one hour, and is designed to be conducted by health professionals who do not specialise in addictions treatment. It is not designed for dependent drinkers, but is most often used with patients who are drinking excessively, and its goal may be to moderate drinking rather than achieve abstinence. Research indicates that brief intervention for alcohol problems is more effective than no intervention, and is often as effective as more extensive intervention.[11]

The key ingredients of brief interventions are summarised by the acronym FRAMES:[8,9]

Feedback: about personal risk or impairment
Responsibility: emphasis on personal responsibility for change
Advice: to cut down or abstain
Menu of strategies: alternative options for changing the drinking pattern
Empathy: listening reflectively without cajoling or confronting
Self-efficacy: interview style to enhance people's belief in their ability to change.

Goal setting, follow-up, and timing have also been identified as important to the effectiveness of brief intervention.

Case study 6.1 continued

You see Ms Quaff fortnightly for the next six weeks, and you learn that her father was an alcoholic. Ms Quaff finds it hard to control her drinking. She realises that she had been colluding with herself for years and that her drinking had caused her many problems.

She drops into your surgery about six months later. She has lost two stone in weight, looks 10 years younger and has changed her job. She has decided that she didn't trust herself to control her drinking and has actually abstained completely. Her blood pressure is now normal and you offer to repeat her blood tests for her.

Collecting data to demonstrate your learning, competence, performance and standards of service delivery

Example cycle of evidence 6.1

- Focus: management of alcohol misuse
- Other relevant foci: prescribing interactions; refusal of tests

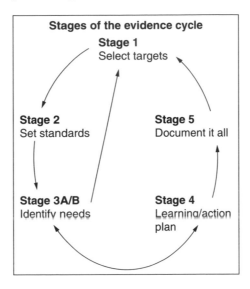

Stages of the evidence cycle

Stage 1
Select targets

Stage 2
Set standards

Stage 5
Document it all

Stage 3A/B
Identify needs

Stage 4
Learning/action plan

Case study 6.2

Ms Barr has returned to see you about her continuing depression. This is her second consultation, one month after being started on an antidepressant drug. The GP had started her on treatment then and had noted in her records that she smelt of alcohol at the morning appointment, and requested blood tests to investigate (full blood count including MCV and liver function tests). Her blood results are not back and you find that she did not actually arrange for her blood to be taken. 'What was the point – I know I am drinking too much, I don't need any tests to tell me that!' Ms Barr feels a little better for taking her anti-depressants, she is sleeping longer in the morning and is less weepy, but still basically depressed. She asks you to examine her swollen and cut knees while she is there – a result of a fall down some stairs. You try to discuss exactly how much alcohol she is drinking and to find out how dependent she is on alcohol by asking the CAGE questions.[12] You wonder how to proceed with someone who does not want to accept help for her admitted problem with alcohol and whether it is safe to continue the antidepressant drug without knowing her liver function.

This is just an example. Keep your task simple. You could choose three or four cycles of evidence to demonstrate your competence each year.

Stage 1: Select your aspirations for good practice

The excellent nurse:

- respects the right of patients to refuse treatments or tests
- is up to date with developments in clinical practice
- chooses specialists to meet the needs of individual patients.

Stage 2: Set the standards for your outcomes

Outcomes might include:

- the way learning is applied
- a learnt skill
- a protocol
- a strategy that is implemented
- meeting recommended standards.

- Have an agreed practice protocol describing the team management of alcohol misuse.
- Become the clinical lead in the practice for patients who misuse alcohol.

Stage 3A: Identify your learning needs

- Chat on the phone with the community psychiatric nurse (CPN) who specialises in helping patients who misuse alcohol, and ask his advice about any techniques for helping people who are not motivated to change. Find out what you 'do not know you do not know'.
- Contact the Primary Care Alcohol Information Service (PCAIS) via the Alcohol Concern website[4] for examples of good practice in tackling alcohol misuse.
- Think about what you know about which drugs are contraindicated where alcohol is known to be misused or liver function is deranged. Look up the contraindications to prescribing a range of antidepressant drugs in the British National Formulary to check your knowledge.[13]

- Talk to other colleagues in the practice about their approach when patients refuse tests or treatment. Find out if you (and they) have learning needs about the legal position.
- Make a list of the symptoms or signs commonly encountered in patients who are misusing alcohol. Compare your list with the World Health Organization document.[3]

Stage 3B: Identify your service needs

> Any of the needs assessment exercises in 3A may also reveal service needs.

- Audit the number of referrals from the practice in last 12 months of patients who misuse alcohol (and other substances) to CPNs or other specialists in the community or in secondary care. How does your referral pattern compare with that of other practices? Could a low referral rate indicate that your practice team is detecting few patients who are abusing alcohol? Alternatively a low referral rate might be because you and colleagues are good at managing such cases in the practice.
- Ask your CPN colleague what services are available for people misusing alcohol for you to refer to or patients to self-refer – are you aware of them all?
- Do you know what you can do to optimise the referral? Find out the extent and type of information about the patient that will help to prioritise referrals. You could discuss this with the CPN to find out if there are other gaps in what you are doing as a practice team.

Stage 4: Make and carry out a learning and action plan

- Read about the management of patients who abuse alcohol. Locate national or local guidelines on the diagnosis and management of alcohol misuse in primary care.[9]
- Attend a health promotion workshop that covers training in motivating patients to change adverse lifestyle habits.
- After obtaining the patient's informed consent, sit in on a consultation of your CPN or psychiatrist specialising in alcohol misuse, with a patient you have referred for help. Watch their approach and learn what else you might have been able to do in your consultation with the patient. Keep a close watch on the patient's progress and outcomes of successive appointments with the specialist.
- Draw up a practice protocol based on what you have learnt about this approach and services from undertaking the learning and service needs assessments. Adapt the national or local guidelines to the setting of your practice.
- Hold an in-house educational session with other nurses and GPs, plus the practice manager, to explain the protocol to the others in your practice team, and gain their ownership. Use the audit of referrals as a focus for any action that needs to be taken.

Stage 5: Document your learning, competence, performance and standards of service delivery

- Include a copy of the new practice protocol.
- Include an anonymised copy of the audit of referrals, the conclusion and any action taken.
- Keep a copy of your notes of the in-house educational session. Comment on the barriers and other issues coming out of the discussion about the protocol, and what you will do as a team to make the protocol work.
- Include a copy of literature for patients to explain how they can get help for problems with alcohol.

Case study 6.2 continued

Ms Barr was able to continue her antidepressant drug, which does not appear to be contraindicated. Two appointments later, Ms Barr is starting to talk to you about her drinking habits. She agrees that she wants to do something about it and does go for her blood tests. Ms Barr also agrees she will go and see a specialist CPN about her addiction to alcohol but she does not attend that appointment.

Example cycle of evidence 6.2

- Focus: managing suspicions of child abuse
- Other relevant foci: deciding to breach patient confidentiality; relationships with patients; teamworking

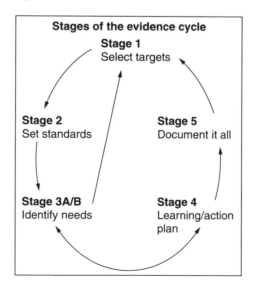

Stages of the evidence cycle

Stage 1
Select targets

Stage 2
Set standards

Stage 5
Document it all

Stage 3A/B
Identify needs

Stage 4
Learning/action plan

> **Case study 6.3**
>
> Mrs Brunt is nursing a swollen eye when she brings in one of her two little girls, Pat, to your health visitor drop-in clinic. After examining Pat's eczema and obtaining a prescription, you ask Mrs Brunt about her eye. It all comes pouring out – her husband's occasional violence after he has had too much to drink (as happened last week), their fear, their debts. Mrs Brunt has almost made up her mind to leave her husband and take the girls with her. She tells you her plans but they seem rather vague. You enquire further about whether their father is ever violent towards the girls, and although Mrs Brunt denies it you have the gut feeling from the reactions of both Mrs Brunt and Pat that the girls are at risk.

This is just an example. Keep your task simple. You could choose three or four cycles of evidence to demonstrate your competence each year.

Stage 1: Select your aspirations for good practice

The excellent nurse:

- acts promptly where child protection is an issue
- makes appropriate judgements about patients who need referral
- respects the patient's right to confidentiality and provides information to colleagues in a manner appropriate to their level of involvement in the patient's care.

Stage 2: Set the standards for your outcomes

Outcomes might include:

- the way learning is applied
- a learnt skill
- a protocol
- a strategy that is implemented
- meeting recommended standards.

- Know when it is good practice to breach patient confidentiality and how to do it.
- Take action in line with local referral protocol and procedures for child protection.

Stage 3A: Identify your learning needs

- Consider what you should do when you have vague suspicions that a child may be at risk of domestic violence or other abuse. Discuss the action you might take with the child protection lead in your primary care organisation (PCO).
- Obtain local protocol and national guidance for child protection and compare what you think you should do with what the protocol states.[14]
- Ring the PCO Caldicott officer to compare what you think and what they recommend about you passing on confidential information to social services (about your suspicions of violence towards Pat Brunt and her sister from their drunken father when you have no evidence).

Stage 3B: Identify your service needs

> Any of the needs assessment exercises in 3A may also reveal service needs.

- Undertake a significant event audit of any incident involving child abuse. Analyse with colleagues whether you and others acted in accordance with best practice protocols or local guidelines.
- Look at the practice protocol about confidentiality and identify the circumstances in which confidential information can be relayed to others without the patient's explicit consent. Compare it with official guidance from your medical defence society or the Department of Health.[15]
- Audit the outcomes of five patients whom you have coded as abusing alcohol. Reflecting on their cases, could more be done in the practice to proactively engage patients in treatment earlier? Could more or different care be provided once those patients have admitted their problems with alcohol?
- If Mr Brunt is registered with the practice, look at his medical records. Search to see if he has an entry about a problem with alcohol and, if so, could the practice team do more? If there is no record of his problem with alcohol, log the information given by his wife and consider if, in retrospect, he has consulted with symptoms and signs that may be attributable to his reported alcohol problem. This might indicate that you or others need to learn to be more alert to the ways in which those who abuse alcohol may present.

Stage 4: Make and carry out a learning and action plan

- Discussions with colleagues (as in Stage 3) will be part of the learning and action plan.
- Reading up on the protocols and guidance described in Stage 3 will form part of your learning plan.
- Attend a workshop on alcoholism.

- Run two in-house educational sessions with your practice team to discuss and formulate action following the results of the significant event analysis (child protection) and audit (patients with problems with alcohol) as described in Stage 3.

Stage 5: Document your learning, competence, performance and standards of service delivery

- Include a reference to the local child protection protocol.
- Include a copy of the booklet describing action professionals should take to safeguard children.[14]
- Record the action plans from the in-house educational discussions of audits, with the repeat audits done or planned for six months later.
- Include an audit of the next case of suspected or proven child abuse occurring in the practice and compare the management with best practice (against the local protocol or national guidance).

Case study 6.3 continued

You ask the healthcare assistant to take Pat to play with a box of toys for a few minutes while you talk privately with her mother. You express your fears about the possibility of Mr Brunt being violent with the children, which she again denies. You discuss your fears with colleagues in the practice and they urge you to contact social services to talk over your concerns, for which you have little evidence. The duty social worker assures you that you have taken the right action and they will investigate the circumstances. Your suspicions prove to be correct, and Pat's older sister does have bruises too from when her Dad lashed out at her the previous week.

The father is not a patient at the practice, so you cannot offer him help with his drinking problem. From what you learn in this exercise, you are much clearer about what action you could have taken.

Example cycle of evidence 6.3

- Focus: relationships with patients
- Other relevant foci: clinical care; health promotion; teaching

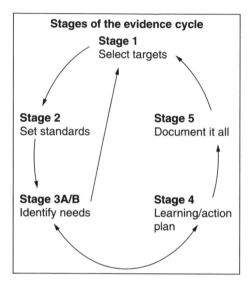

Stages of the evidence cycle

Stage 1 Select targets

Stage 2 Set standards

Stage 5 Document it all

Stage 3A/B Identify needs

Stage 4 Learning/action plan

Case study 6.4

Rocky comes to see you in the university vacation. He is consulting you, the nurse practitioner, at a same-day consultation appointment because of his morning sickness, sweating and, most of all, the tremor of his hands that makes working on the computer keyboard difficult. He is in his third year at university and staying at his parents' home – out in the sticks. You ask him to tell you more about himself. His face lights up as he tells you about the 'wicked' time he has at uni with his mates, out clubbing, doing some lectures but missing others. He cannot wait to get back to uni as he rarely goes out at night when staying at his parents' home, being stuck out in the countryside without transport.

This is just an example. Keep your task simple. You could choose three or four cycles of evidence to demonstrate your competence each year.

Stage 1: Select your aspirations for good practice

The excellent nurse:

- uses clear language appropriate for the patient
- uses investigations when they will help the management of the condition
- promotes a healthy lifestyle to all patients.

Stage 2: Set the standards for your outcomes

Outcomes might include:

- the way learning is applied
- a learnt skill
- a protocol
- a strategy that is implemented
- meeting recommended standards.

- Be able to motivate patients to pursue healthy lifestyles.

Stage 3A: Identify your learning needs

- Seek feedback from patients whom you have advised about their unhealthy lifestyles (poor or fatty diet, lack of exercise, smoking, excessive alcohol). Focus on the clarity of information you gave or your way of giving it (your teaching skills).
- Seek feedback from colleagues about your ability to motivate patients with unhealthy lifestyles. Ask them to record their impressions when they have seen the same patients on subsequent occasions.
- Undertake an audit of 10 consecutive patients whom you have advised to stop smoking, lose weight, take up exercise, cut down or stop drinking alcohol. Follow them over time to see the results of your (and others') advice giving, by reviewing their notes one year later or asking them directly 6–12 months later when they consult you for the same or different conditions.

Stage 3B: Identify your service needs

Any of the needs assessment exercises in 3A may also reveal service needs.

- Review all the literature that exists in the practice for advising patients who abuse alcohol or have a drinking problem. Is it current, clear, and relevant for different age groups? Ask patients of different age groups to 'proof read' them and comment on the way information is given.

- Undertake an audit of 50 patients whose age ranges from 16–24 years, to ascertain for how many you as a practice have recorded lifestyle details, including alcohol consumption. Also record what action or advice was given subsequently for any who were drinking more alcohol than is recommended for a healthy lifestyle.
- Draw up a patient pathway for a person like Rocky. Start from the first consultation with an alcohol-related symptom or sign and what investigations, treatment and advice should be offered. Discuss the pathway as a practice team to add in other alternative approaches that colleagues take and review how much similarity there is between individual team members.

Stage 4: Make and carry out a learning and action plan

- Attend a seminar run by health promotion to learn more about motivating patients. Establish how to maximise your impact if they are either not contemplating or are contemplating changing their lifestyles.
- Sit in on sessions with a colleague who has good track record in motivating others to change their lifestyle e.g. in a structured smoking cessation session, and learn what you can apply in the approaches you take to patients.
- Invite that expert colleague to critique your approach in a follow-up session with a patient you are trying to motivate to change their lifestyle (e.g. with the patient's permission for sitting in, or from an audiotape), and discuss your performance together.
- Run a focus group of young people to discuss the patient literature and how the practice might improve services, especially to help them attain healthy lifestyles. Involve others who might help develop improved services e.g. from a local leisure centre, youth club, etc.
- Write a protocol for yourself and the practice team on helping patients to attain a healthy lifestyle, including when liver function tests, full blood count, fasting lipids should be undertaken.

Stage 5: Document your learning, competence, performance and standards of service delivery

- Keep a copy of the practice protocol with the indications for blood tests and the action needed.
- Keep a copy of the audit and action and learning undertaken as a result.
- Keep the revised practice literature and links to leisure and youth services following the focus group meeting.
- Make a record of your reflections on what you have learnt about motivation techniques, from sitting in and the follow-up discussions with your expert colleague.
- Repeat the audit of 10 consecutive patients to demonstrate your improved skills in motivating people to switch to healthier lifestyles.

Case study 6.4 continued

Rocky is surprised and shocked that you think he is exhibiting symptoms of withdrawal from alcohol, as he had never considered it. He does not want to talk about it and rushes off. You see him again when he consults about his acne, six months later when he has finished his degree and moved back to the local area, in a flat with his friends. He tells you that he has really thought through how much alcohol he was drinking and realises that you were probably right. Since then he has not drunk alcohol when on his own – it was automatic before to have cans stashed around his bedroom. He has gone out less with his mates and although he still binges on alcohol at times, it is less often and he is gradually cutting down.

References

1   UK Alcohol Forum (1997) *Guidelines for the Management of Alcohol Problems in Primary Care and General Psychiatry*. Tangent Medical Education, London.

2   Waller S, Naidoo B and Thom B (2002) *Prevention and Reduction of Alcohol Misuse. Evidence Briefing*. NHS Health Development Agency, London.

3   Babor TF, Higgins-Biddle JC, Saunders JB and Monteiro MG (2001) *The Alcohol Use Disorders Identification Test. World Health Organization*, Geneva. http://whqlibdoc.who.int/hq/2001/WHO_MSD_MSB_01.6a.pdf

4   Alcohol Concern: www.alcoholconcern.org.uk (accessed 27 April 2005)

5   Royal College of Physicians (1987) *A Great and Growing Evil – the medical consequences of alcohol abuse*. Royal College of Physicians, London.

6   Greenfield TK (2001) Individual risk of alcohol related disease and problems. In: N Heather, TJ Peters and T Stockwell (eds) *International Handbook of Alcohol Dependence and Problems*. Wiley, London. www.dfc.unifi.it/sia/alcohoandhealth.pdf (accessed 27 April 2005)

7   www.acad.org.uk/04.html (accessed 27 April 2005)

8   Bien TH, Miller WR and Tonigan JS (1993) Brief interventions for alcohol problems: a review. *Addiction*. **88**: 315–36.

9   Wallace PG and Haines AP (1984) General practitioner and health promotion: what patients think. *British Medical Journal*. **289**: 534–6.

10 Wilk AI, Jensen NM and Havighurst TC (1997) Meta-analysis of randomised controlled trials addressing brief interventions in heavy alcohol drinkers. *Journal of General Internal Medicine*. **12**: 274–83.

11 Edwards G, Orford J, Egert S *et al*. (1997) Alcoholism: a controlled trial of 'treatment' and 'advice'. *Journal of Studies on Alcohol*. **38**: 1004–31.

12 www.netdoctor.co.uk/health_advice/facts/alcoholism.htm (accessed 27 April 2005)

13 Joint Formulary Committee (2005) *British National Formulary*. British Medical Association and Royal Pharmaceutical Society of Great Britain, London. www.bnf.org

14   Department of Health (2003) *What to Do If You're Worried a Child is being Abused.* HMSO, London. www.dh.gov.uk/assetRoot/04/06/13/03/04061303.pdf (accessed 27 April 2005)

15   Department of Health (2003) *Confidentiality. NHS Code of Practice.* Department of Health, London.

Further reading

• Ashworth M and Gerada C (1998) Addiction and dependence-alcohol. In: T Davies and TK Craig (eds) *ABC of Mental Health.* BMJ Publications, London.
• Deehan A, Marshall EJ and Strang J (1998) Tackling alcohol misuse: opportunities and obstacles in primary care. *British Journal of General Practice.* **48**: 1779–82.
• Fleeman ND (1997) Alcohol home detoxification: a literature review. *Alcohol and Alcoholism.* **32**: 649–56.
• Hartz C, Plant M and Watts M (1990) *Alcohol and Health – a handbook for nurses, midwives and health visitors.* The Medical Council on Alcoholism, London.
• Managing the heavy drinker in primary care (2000) *Drug and Therapeutics Bulletin.* **3**: 60–4.

7

Palliative care

Nurses frequently take a lead role in the management of chronic diseases or long-term conditions. Please reread the introduction to Chapter 4 about your need to be qualified for a specialist role or that of community matron.

Case study 7.1

Nurse Jolly, a new staff nurse on the community, brings some difficult cases to you as his mentor. The common theme is that the patients are being cared for at home with an illness from which they are not expected to recover. He is finding it difficult to cope with his own feelings and with the teamworking necessary for the control of symptoms. He comments that he feels like a spare part, just relaying suggestions from the palliative care nurse.

What issues you should cover

Palliative care is the support of people who are suffering from an illness from which no cure can be anticipated. Where possible, palliative care is delivered where the person wants to be. Usually it can be provided in a combination of:

- the person's own home
- a hospice
- a hospital
- a nursing home.

Family, relatives and friends are usually the main carers. Professional help comes from a team and is not just concerned with the relief of symptoms in people suffering from cancer, although it is often thought of in this narrow sense. The aim of palliative care is to maximise the quality of the person's life. Physical, emotional, social and spiritual needs may need attention. Meeting the individual needs of the person being cared for, and the caregivers, is a team effort that co-ordinates and delivers a range of services (*see* Figure 7.1).

Consider how information can be transferred from one carer to another. The individual being looked after, or his/her main carer, may not have the skills or knowledge to pass on details to others in the team of treatment or arrangements being made. Some patients and their carers like to keep a personal record of what is happening and what needs to be done. In most cases, the care plan and nursing

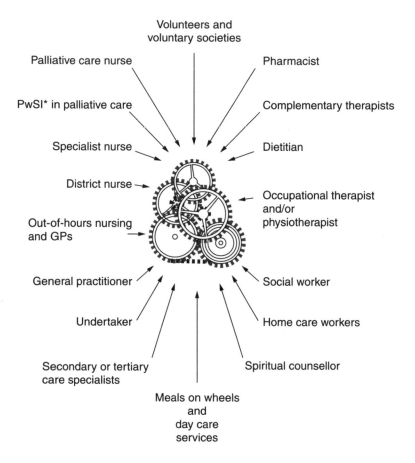

Palliative care nurse

PwSI* in palliative care

Specialist nurse

District nurse

Out-of-hours nursing
and GPs

General practitioner

Undertaker

Secondary or tertiary
care specialists

Volunteers and
voluntary societies

Pharmacist

Complementary therapists

Dietitian

Occupational therapist
and/or
physiotherapist

Social worker

Home care workers

Spiritual counsellor

Meals on wheels
and
day care
services

*Practitioner with special interest.

Figure 7.1:   Some team members in palliative care.

notes, kept with the patient, are the best record of what treatment and plans are being made. Nurse Jolly should make a point of reading these and recording (and signing legibly) any changes in condition or arrangements he makes. These records can be invaluable if a stranger has to be involved – perhaps in an emergency at night when a different district nurse or doctor attends.

Treat each person as an individual

To understand the needs of another person, Nurse Jolly must set aside his own beliefs or philosophy. Some concept of basic tenets of other cultures and religions will help him, but he must resist the urge to categorise patients. He has to find out about the expectations, values and beliefs of the person before him, and what emotional, spiritual and practical support is available. Different cultures and religions have varying degrees of adherence and influence amongst communities. Sometimes there are different practices depending upon the country of origin of the individual or that of their family. As always, it is important to ask the person and those close to the sufferer. Dignity in palliative care involves information and good communication, pain control, alleviation of distressing symptoms and support as well as social care, spiritual care, psychological support and bereavement care. Anxiety, fear and hopelessness will make all other symptoms worse and less easy to manage, so the first task is to start from the standpoint of the sufferer and their carers, and help them to make some sense of what is happening. Giving information or helping people find the information they need, at a suitable pace, is a skill to be learnt. Knowing where to look for information can be the first step. Charitable organisations and patient groups can be immensely supportive and an accessible website giving links to many other sources of help and guidance can be a useful resource for many patients, carers and professionals.[1]

Meetings with the patient and the carers to discuss what is needed, and whether the expectations for continuing help at home are being met, help to keep everyone on course for the smooth running of care. Regrettably, the lack of resources may mean that someone cannot be cared for at home as they wish, because of lack of, or delays in, sorting out benefits, equipment (such as hoists, bath aids, wheelchairs), or people who can help. The recommendations for a modern service for people with cancer (*see* Box 7.1),[2] and the various guidelines for people with cancer from the National Institute for Clinical Excellence (NICE),[3] including the *Guidance on Improving Supportive and Palliative Care for Adults with Cancer*, may help Nurse Jolly know what the standard of service should be.

Nurse Jolly may find that referral to a palliative care specialist nurse has already been made by someone at the hospital before discharge home. If not, he may have to broach the subject himself and explore sensitively how someone would accept such referral. Many people believe that referral to a hospice, or for assessment by the community palliative care nurse, means that they are about to die. It is important to emphasise the support and specialist knowledge about relief of symptoms, provision of benefits, equipment and access to voluntary and professional help that the palliative care service can provide. After a referral, a community-based specialist nurse, usually a Macmillan nurse if the patient has cancer,[4] will assess the whole situation. Macmillan Cancer Relief helps provide expert care and practical support. They fund specialist Macmillan nurses, doctors and other health professionals, and provide cancer care centres and hospices. They provide a range of information and support services, including the Macmillan CancerLine (the telephone helpline[4]), useful publications and local cancer information centres. They support local self-help groups and advise on, and sometimes give, financial support. They liaise with other professionals such as physiotherapists, occupational therapists and complementary therapists to provide the most appropriate care for the patient.

Macmillan nurses usually act in an advisory capacity but Marie Curie nurses are available in some areas to provide free nursing care. Marie Curie nurses now care for almost half of all cancer patients who die at home in the UK. They work through the night or during the day to provide one-on-one care for the patient and provide practical and emotional support for families at what can be an exhausting time.[1] In other areas, district nurse services, stretched at the best of times, have to be supplemented by volunteers, relatives or paid agency nurses.

If nursing care is not required, social services are asked to carry out a needs assessment and put into place means tested assistance, such as home care or meals on wheels. A social worker will also be able to help with applications for benefits. Nurse Jolly needs to be aware of a 'DS1500'. The DS1500 is a form designed to speed up the payment of the Disability Living Allowance, Attendance Allowance or Incapacity Benefit. It is usually issued under special rules, after prior request by the patient or their carer or at the suggestion of any primary care team member. The GP or a hospital consultant can complete the DS1500. It is usually issued when the patient is considered to be approaching the terminal stage of their disease. In Social Security law, a patient is terminally ill if they are suffering from a progressive disease and are not expected to live longer than six months. The timing is, of course, very difficult to judge, but the decision to issue is one for the clinician involved, who would then be able to justify their decision.

Box 7.1:   Gold Standards Framework (GSF)[2]

The Gold Standards Framework (GSF) is a practice-based system to improve the organisation and quality of palliative care services for patients who are at home in their last year of life. This practical framework is based on seven 'gold' standards which relate to teamwork and continuity of care, advanced planning, symptom control and support of patients/carers, and include:

- *communication*: maintaining a supportive care register
- *co-ordination*: a nominated co-ordinator for palliative care within the practice (e.g. district nurse)
- *control of symptoms*: regular assessment of symptoms from the patient's perspective
- *continuity* (out of hours): transfer of information to out-of-hours services
- *continued learning*: learning is clinical, organisational/strategic and attitudes/approaches (e.g. communication skills)
- *carer support*: carers are supported emotionally, practically and in bereavement
- *care in the dying phase*: terminal care is appropriate and follows an integrated care pathway approach.

If the patient has a condition other than cancer, such as chronic obstructive pulmonary disease, Nurse Jolly may need to find out how to contact relevant support services. The genitourinary medicine department usually organises the relevant specialist services for patients with acquired immunodeficiency syndrome (AIDS). Outreach specialist nurses may be available for particular conditions, but availability tends to be very variable from area to area. In a few areas, there is a common care pathway for any palliative care, but it is more common for it to be fragmented between departments and organisations. A practice resource list can help patients, carers and health professionals to contact the relevant sources of care and support.

Relief of symptoms

Nurse Jolly should look at the patient's prescribed medication to see if it is still relevant and discuss it with the GP. It is often forgotten that medication may be prescribed to prevent events happening in the future e.g. treatment for hypertension, or to reduce cholesterol levels, which becomes irrelevant and unnecessary when the life expectancy is short. Previously prescribed medication may be contraindicated with the changes in treatment now required.

Pain

Nurse Jolly should remember that not all pain is related to the primary condition – it may be secondary to the treatment – e.g. constipation due to opiates, gout precipitated by diuretics, or scar tissue after radiotherapy. It may be coincidental such as with migraine or osteoarthritis. Any perception of pain will be influenced by fear, loneliness, boredom, depression, previous experience of ill-health and individual attitudes.

Cancer pain is continuous, so it should be treated all the time, not just when it emerges. He should discuss the nature of chronic pain with patients who often believe that chronic pain is the same as acute pain only present all the time. Explain that acute pain is a danger signal that something is wrong. Chronic pain tells you that something has been wrong in the past and the nerves have become used to passing that signal onto the brain. Many people are unwilling to take adequate pain relief for chronic pain because they think they will not be able to receive acute pain warning signals. They need to be aware that they can relieve chronic pain with analgesics but still be able to feel the acute pain of, for example, cutting themselves on the edge of tin, or pulling a muscle during over-exertion. Beliefs about how chronic pain happens often lead people into inactivity. They avoid anything that might cause the pain in the short term instead of increasing their activity to improve muscle strength and co-ordination and stretch tight scar tissue to decrease the pain in the long term. Taking enough pain relief to prevent the emergence of pain, that is prophylactically and not just in response to pain, reduces the passage of the pain messages along the nerves and helps to prevent the nerves becoming 'accustomed to passing that message'. Established pain leads to structural and neurochemical changes in the central nervous system that consolidate the pattern of pain. Taking enough pain relief also permits the graduated and frequent activity that improves chronic pain.

Cancer-related pain may be:

- soft-tissue or visceral pain and respond to paracetamol and opiates
- bone pain that can respond partially to paracetamol and opiates, or to non-steroidal anti-inflammatory drugs (NSAIDs), or be relieved by radiotherapy
- nerve-affected or nerve-mediated, requiring drugs that act on the nervous system
- related to the impact of a cancer on adjacent tissues, e.g. in raised intracranial pressure or abdominal masses.

Most people in the UK prefer oral medications, but consider with patients what would suit them best. There is increasing acceptance of transdermal application via a skin patch, although it may take some time to initially establish the right dose by titration. Some patients prefer suppositories if they have nausea or disturbed nights, because of break-through pain after shorter-acting oral medication. Paracetamol and opiates are generally used in a 'ladder' (see Box 7.2), increasing the dose of opiates until the pain is under control. Opiates also suppress cough and relieve breathlessness. Psychological techniques, such as cognitive therapy, can help patients to learn to manage their pain better, and other techniques such as self-hypnosis or acupuncture may be helpful for some individuals.

Box 7.2:   Analgesic ladder

Start here:
Non-opiate e.g. paracetamol

Weak opiate e.g. codeine plus paracetamol: add medication to prevent constipation as soon as an opiate is added

Strong opiate e.g. morphine plus non-opioid or fentanyl patch (*see British National Formulary*[5] for equivalent strength to morphine), e.g.:

- start with oral morphine 10 mg 4 hourly (i.e. six times a day)
- increase by a third to half every 3–5 days according to response
- transfer to the same dose of slow release morphine every 12 h (or a patch), with standard release morphine available for break-through pain or increases as required.

Other medications that can help to control pain are listed in Table 7.1.

Nurse Jolly should anticipate the common problems when introducing opiates. A stimulant laxative should be added as soon as an opiate is started and the dose increased when the opiate strength is increased. A softening or bulking agent alone is rarely successful. Sleepiness is usual when starting each dose increment and then wears off. Nausea is also common (see Table 7.2 p.125). Other problems can include a dry mouth, itching, sweating, hallucinations and myoclonic jerks. Although tolerance

Table 7.1: Additional medication to control non-opiate-sensitive pain[6]

Type of pain	Medication	Considerations
Bone pain; pleuritic pain; soft tissue infiltration	NSAIDs; consider radiotherapy	Avoid NSAIDs if a previous history of GI ulceration. Selective Cox II inhibitors reduce but do not completely avoid risks of GI upset and damage. NSAIDs can be given with a proton pump inhibitor e.g. lansoprozole
Raised intracranial pressure; enlarged liver or spleen; enlarging tumours	Steroids; consider radiotherapy	Dexametasone usually used (2 mg dexametasone = 15 mg prednisolone). Gastroprotection also required as for NSAIDs
Nerve-related pain e.g. shooting, stabbing or burning	Amitriptyline	Used in lower doses than for depression, start low and increase to reduce sedation and dry mouth
	Carbamazepine, gabapentin	Higher dose use may be limited by the side-effects
Root pain	Steroids, trancutaneous electrical nerve stimulation (TENS machine), consider nerve block	A loan of a TENS machine can usually be arranged
Muscle spasm	Diazepam	May cause sedation but can also relieve anxiety
	Baclofen	Increase dose slowly to avoid sedation and muscle hypotonia
Tenesmus	As for nerve-related pain Chlorpromazine	Sedation a problem but useful if restlessness is also present
	Nifedipine	Increase dose slowly to avoid flushing

may occur, increases in dose are usually required for advancing disease. Always look at other causes for pain break-through.

Constipation

Exclude constipation as the cause of agitation and distress before requesting the addition of other drugs. Clinical examination should include abdominal and rectal examination. Never forget that uncontrolled diarrhoea may be overflow liquid finding its way past a valve-like effect of hard faeces. A good first choice for the prevention of opiate-induced or inactivity constipation is a combination of a stimulant laxative together with a softening agent, e.g. co-danthrusate, co-danthramer, or senna with lactulose.[6,7] If prescribed co-danthrusate or co-danthramer, alert the patient to the fact that their urine may become discoloured and red. High doses of lactulose can cause flatulence and abdominal cramps. Relatively high doses of laxative may be needed. Tailor your treatment of existing constipation according to your clinical findings:

- rectum full of hard faeces: lubricate with glycerin suppositories or an oil enema, then use a stimulant laxative with or without a softener
- rectum full of soft faeces: use a stimulant laxative which will take about 10 h to work
- rectum still full after the above treatment: manual evacuation, perhaps with sedation or an anxiolytic
- rectum empty: consider if obstruction is present or high constipation
- loaded colon with colic: start a softener, e.g. docusate
- loaded colon without colic: try a stimulant laxative.

Nausea and/or vomiting

Constipation may be accompanied by nausea, or nausea may be present alone with or without vomiting. Useful medications are listed in Table 7.2.

Using drugs in a syringe driver

The syringe driver is a small, portable, battery-driven infusion pump, used to give medication subcutaneously via a syringe, usually over 24 hours. It is a useful alternative if gastric symptoms are a persistent problem despite medication, or if the patient prefers not to have medication orally. Diamorphine is the opiate of choice for subcutaneous infusion because of its high solubility. It also helps with breathlessness. Divide the dose of morphine by three to convert from morphine to diamorphine. Other drugs can be added to the syringe driver (*see* Table 7.2). Midazolam can be added to control restlessness, myoclonic jerks or as an anticonvulsant if required. The syringe driver needs to be checked regularly for irritation at the injection site, crystallisation of the drugs, leakage, correct volume remaining and that the battery is not exhausted. Drugs used in the syringe driver may be used outside their product licence, so keep meticulous records. It is good practice to use as few drugs as possible in the syringe driver, usually only one or two, as data on compatibility are sparse. Water for injection is usually used as the diluent, as physiological saline may cause precipitation when more than one drug is used.[5] For a more comprehensive guide to syringe driver use refer to the *Palliative Care Formulary*.[7]

Table 7.2: Some drugs for nausea and vomiting.[6] Consult the *British National Formulary*[5] for others less commonly used

Drug and action	Other indications	Characteristics	Cautions
Metoclopropamide[a]: increases peristalsis in upper gut; dopamine antagonist		Oral tablets or liquid; intramuscular injection	Extrapyramidal effects especially in children or young people
Domperidone: increases peristalsis in upper gut; dopamine antagonist		Oral tablets or liquid; suppositories	Less likely to cause dystonia
Cyclizine[a]: acts on vestibular and vomiting centres	Vertigo	Oral tablets; intramuscular, intravenous injection	Drowsiness; caution in severe heart failure
Haloperidol[a]: blocks dopamine receptors at chemoreceptor trigger zone	Hiccups; psychotic symptoms; agitation	Oral tablets; intramuscular, intravenous injection	Dry mouth; hypotension; extrapyramidal symptoms
Levomeprazine[a]: blocks dopamine and serotonin receptors, also acts at vestibular and vomiting centres	Psychotic symptoms; adjunct for pain; agitation	Oral tablets; intramuscular, intravenous injection	Postural hypotension; sedation
Ondansetron[a], **granisetron**: block 5-HT$_3$ receptors	Especially for nausea and vomiting induced by chemotherapy	Oral tablets; intramuscular, intravenous injection. Ondansetron also in suppositories	Constipation, flushing and rash
Dexametasone[a]: reduces inflammatory oedema, central and peripheral anti-emetic effects	Pain relief	Oral tablets; intramuscular, intravenous injection	Steroid side-effects
Hyoscine hydrobromide[a]: reduces GI secretions and motility	Excessive respiratory secretions; motion sickness	Oral tablets; patch; intramuscular injection	Closed angle glaucoma; urinary retention; GI obstruction
Octreotide[a]; **lanreotide**[a]: reduce GI secretions and motility	Relief of symptoms from neuroendocrine tumours; variceal bleeding	Subcutaneous injection	Affects diabetic control

[a]Also useful in a syringe driver as a subcutaneous infusion

Complementary therapies[8]

Acupuncture is often used successfully for both pain relief and treatment of nausea. Surveys of the available scientific research into acupuncture suggest that it is definitely an effective treatment for nausea caused by chemotherapy when treating cancer.[8]

Aromatherapy may help with relaxation and feelings of improved wellbeing. Particularly when combined with massage, the close physical contact and the relationship with a therapist can help to increase people's sense of being cared for. Caution is required where essential oils are used that may affect skin that is already sensitive following radiotherapy.

Hypnotherapy may be used as an adjunct to other therapy and has been shown to ameliorate some psychological and medical conditions. It can be used together with therapies such as cognitive behavioural therapy to enable patients to view their illness in a less negative or catastrophic way.[8]

Over-the-counter herbal therapies should not be taken. Always ask about any herbal remedies or supplements as they may be contraindicated unless prescribed by a medical herbalist with full knowledge of the conventional medication being taken.[9] Many herbal remedies interact with medication e.g. St John's Wort with medication for AIDS or ginger with warfarin. Some may be contraindicated in certain cancers, e.g. echinacea in lymphoma.[10]

Other complementary therapies, e.g. Reiki, head massage, spiritual healing, may also be offered by the local hospice or obtained elsewhere by patients and their carers. Benefits of improved symptom control, quality of life and patient satisfaction have been demonstrated, but various questions remain. The quality of evidence for many of these therapies is poor and it is not known if the specific techniques are as important as their shared 'holistic' context. The lack of evidence about the way in which therapies work also obscures any possible unwanted effects. Although many of the therapies make patients feel better, claims for improvements to survival from cancer may give false hope.[8]

Dry mouth

A dry mouth is a distressing and frequent problem. Good mouth care, sucking ice or pineapple chunks or artificial saliva may help. Take swabs for thrush if suspected – it may just look red and shiny, not with the classic white patches – and if confirmed, treat with antifungal preparations, e.g. nystatin, miconazole or amphotericin.[5] Bacterial or viral infections should be treated, and malignant ulcers are often infected with anaerobic bacteria causing a foul smell. Treat anaerobic infections with metronidazole orally, rectally or as a gel.[5]

Distress

Perhaps the most important treatment is for people to spend time with the patient – to appreciate with the patient what life was like before, to acknowledge the person that remains despite the illness and disability, and to show care for the patient and the carers, discussing what would help to make life more comfortable or bearable.

Sometimes it is more important for patients to be able to talk than to have drug treatment for their symptoms. Some patients become more agitated and distressed when they do not feel in control of their mental functions because of inappropriate sedation.

Giving bad news is a skill that is difficult to acquire.[11] Always check with patients that what they have heard you say is what you mean – health professionals often use words that patients/relatives/carers do not understand, even when they are trying to explain things clearly. Also, consider the response of the individual – it will always be different from the last person you talked to about similar bad news. Go at the pace of the patient and always establish what they already know, or think they know, before giving any more information. Health professionals have to talk, not just about the illness, but also about the treatments, the need for tests, and about the uncertainty of the future. Such details may need to be repeated because of the difficulties in taking in information when emotionally upset. Anger, guilt and blame are common reactions people have to bad news. These emotions need understanding and discussion, so that the emotion is not directed towards inappropriate targets, such as blaming them-selves, health professionals or their god.

Nurse Jolly will have his own feelings to cope with as well. Identification with the emotions of the patient and carers and feelings of failure are common. Denial is a common mechanism for coping, and may lead to collusion not to mention the seriousness of the condition. Denial is rarely complete and Nurse Jolly can use the same open-ended questions that he employs in his everyday consultations, e.g. 'I wonder how it looks to you?' Nurse Jolly may want to consider attending a course to help him with this type of problem,[11] or just generally improve his communication skills.

Emergencies

Nurse Jolly should think about how to avoid emergencies, especially as these often result in a patient having an otherwise avoidable hospital admission. These include:

- hypercalcaemia
- bone fractures
- superior vena caval obstruction
- spinal cord compression
- epileptic seizures
- haemorrhage.

Hypercalcaemia occurs in 40–50% of people with multiple myeloma and breast cancer, less often in other cancers.[6] Treatment of hypercalcaemia can markedly improve the patient's symptoms even when the disease is advanced. In mild hypercalcaemia, patients have symptoms of nausea, anorexia and vomiting, with thirst, polyuria and constipation – non-specific symptoms common in terminal care – so Nurse Jolly needs to think about it and be prepared to check serum calcium. More severe symptoms include dehydration, drowsiness, confusion and coma, and cardiac arrhythmias. The corrected calcium level is calculated with the value for serum albumin, so this also needs to be checked, together with urea and electrolytes in case an intravenous infusion is required. Saline for rehydration may be followed by a biphosphonate infusion.[6] Treatment with biphosphonates usually corrects the serum calcium in 80% of patients within a week. Treatment of the underlying cancer may prevent recurrence, but if not, oral biphosphonates or infusions every three weeks may be needed.

Bone fractures may be prevented by oral biphosphonates, but they may still occur in osteoporosis, metastatic osteolytic deposits or secondary to trauma. Appropriate treatment depends on the general state of the patient, but may include fixation or radiotherapy.

The symptoms of obstruction of the vena cava are very frightening, with severe breathlessness and a sensation of drowning. Other symptoms include swelling of the face, especially around the eyes, neck and arms. The patient may complain of visual changes, headache, dizziness and fainting. Give immediate treatment with small doses of opiates e.g. 5 mg every four hours if not already receiving an opiate, with or without diazepam. High-dose corticosteroids (dexametasone 16 mg/day) can usually be reduced after the first five days, and referral for radiotherapy discussed.

Spinal cord compression may be gradual and difficult to spot in its early stages. Weakness of the legs is often attributed to the general state of debility, and urinary or bowel problems to the medication. Nurse Jolly needs to think of spinal cord compression in any patient with cancer who complains of back pain, especially if any neurological signs are also present. A magnetic resonance scan can localise any areas of compression and allow targeted radiotherapy.

A patient who has a brain tumour or secondary deposits may need an anticonvulsant. If oral medication is discontinued then Nurse Jolly should anticipate the need for alternative delivery of anticonvulsant medication e.g. midazolam 30 mg/24 h via a syringe driver, or rectal diazepam (10 mg).

If the patient is coughing up blood, Nurse Jolly needs to establish where the bleeding originates – the chest, nose, upper respiratory tract or even the gastrointestinal tract. Bleeding may need to be controlled by radiotherapy or laser therapy. In the last few hours of life, haemoptysis, haematemesis or erosion of a major blood vessel may cause distressing loss of blood. He should make sure that medication is available so that an injection (intravenously if there is circulatory shut-down) of an opiate and diazepam can help to reduce awareness and fear in the patient. Anticipation and preparation help to reduce the distress of carers, and the use of green or dark-coloured towels reduces the visual impact.

Case study 7.1 continued

After the mentorship session, Nurse Jolly draws up a plan to meet some of his learning needs. In the process of helping him meet some of these from the practice resources and elsewhere, you learn quite a bit as well! He begins to feel more competent and able to be proactive in some suggestions for meeting the needs of patients who require palliative care. He finds talking to the palliative care nurse helps him to understand how he might learn to cope with his emotional responses, and is relieved to find that that other professionals suffer from doubts and difficulties as well.

Collecting data to demonstrate your learning, competence, performance and standards of service delivery

Example cycle of evidence 7.1

- Focus: relationships with patients
- Other relevant foci: clinical care; working with colleagues

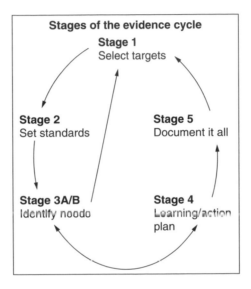

Stages of the evidence cycle

Stage 1
Select targets

Stage 2
Set standards

Stage 5
Document it all

Stage 3A/B
Identify needs

Stage 4
Learning/action plan

Case study 7.2

Mrs Ovum had been admitted to hospital urgently with a large pleural effusion and after many tests disseminated ovarian cancer had been diagnosed. She was discharged home after a course of chemotherapy and has asked for a home visit. The GP has asked you to make contact with Mrs Ovum, so you can start building a relationship as the district nurse providing palliative care. When you arrive her mother lets you in and whispers to you in the hallway: 'She doesn't know what is wrong with her. She thinks she has had treatment for an ovarian cyst'. Her husband is also there, while her father has taken the children out for a while. Mrs Ovum asks you to explain what she has had done at the hospital and says that she cannot understand why she feels so tired. You can tell by the non-verbal signals and anxious looks of her relatives that you could easily say the wrong thing.

This is just an example. Keep your task simple. You could choose three or four cycles of evidence to demonstrate your competence each year.

Stage 1: Select your aspirations for good practice

The excellent nurse:

- is up to date with developments in clinical practice and regularly reviews his or her knowledge and performance
- is guided by the patient in revealing information about the amount and nature of information that he/she wishes to have.

Stage 2: Set the standards for your outcomes

Outcomes might include:

- the way learning is applied
- a learnt skill
- a protocol
- a strategy that is implemented
- meeting recommended standards.

- A comprehensive source of information about terminal conditions is available to members of the practice team.
- Team members caring for someone who is terminally ill communicate to each other their actions and the information given to patients.

Stage 3A: Identify your learning needs

- Establish whether you know how to find information about specific cancer treatments or patient support organisations.
- Self-assess how much you know about how and what to tell patients about their terminal condition.
- Reflect on how you manage the conflict between telling the truth and protecting patients from psychological distress.

Stage 3B: Identify your service needs

> Any of the needs assessment exercises in 3A may also reveal service needs.

- Audit the records of three patients with terminal conditions to identify any gaps in communication between team members.
- Review the length of time patients with terminal conditions are waiting for treatment by others or for equipment e.g. by an occupational therapist, for a commode, or for a TENS machine, and the waiting time for an initial appointment with a palliative care nurse. Consider what you might have done to speed any of these processes, including supplying evidence to your PCO to influence the commissioning process.

Stage 4: Make and carry out a learning and action plan

- Read information about investigations into how patients are told about a terminal diagnosis.[11,12]
- Look up information about ovarian cancer so that you know enough to discuss it if necessary.[13]
- Attend a workshop examining the ethical and practical dilemmas of managing patients with terminal illnesses.
- Run an educational session at the practice for the practice primary healthcare team, including GPs, practice nurses, attached physiotherapist, district nursing colleagues, the palliative care nurse and any others with an interest, to share patients' views and the results of your audit on the difficulties and gaps in communication. Present the draft treatment policy for discussion, before accepting it as a practice team.
- Discuss how the agreed treatment policy can be implemented with key people in the practice team, and decide what shortfalls there are in terms of resources (e.g. availability of equipment or therapy or over-long referral routes) and liaise with the PCO about unmet needs.

Stage 5: Document your learning, competence, performance and standards of service delivery

- Your reflective diary comments about how you manage the conflict between telling the truth and protecting patients from psychological distress and what you can put into practice from the workshop.
- Keep notes on best practice and ovarian cancer from your information search.
- Include a copy of the agreed practice policy for communication between team members caring for someone who is receiving palliative care.
- Include a copy of the letter to the PCO detailing shortfalls in provision for palliative care.
- Include the letter of thanks you receive from Mrs Ovum's mother for your help.

Case study 7.2 continued

You ask Mrs Ovum what she knows about her condition. She says that she had a large ovarian cyst that was causing pressure on her lungs and she has had chemotherapy to shrink the cyst, as it could not be removed. You talk about the side-effects of chemotherapy and how tired that can make someone feel. She seems happier at this information and you ask her to write down any questions she thinks of after your visit and you can discuss them next time. You resolve to look up information about ovarian cancer so that you are better prepared if Mrs Ovum asks you outright about ovarian cancer.[1,12] On the way out, her mother tries to impress on you that you must not tell Mrs Ovum that she has cancer. You acknowledge and comfort her about her own distress about her daughter's illness. You tell her that many patients with cancer know that they have it, but do not want to discuss it. You say to Mrs Ovum's mother that you will be guided by what Mrs Ovum wants to talk about.

Over the next few weeks, it emerges that Mrs Ovum is aware of her diagnosis but has been trying to hide this from her mother. Many tears are shed when the two of them are able to talk more openly about the future.

Example cycle of evidence 7.2

- Focus: clinical care; palliative care emergencies
- Other relevant focus: relationships with patients; working with colleagues

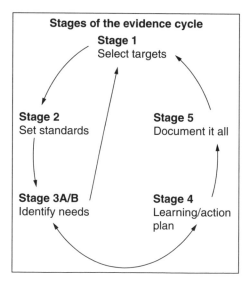

Stages of the evidence cycle

Stage 1
Select targets

Stage 2
Set standards

Stage 5
Document it all

Stage 3A/B
Identify needs

Stage 4
Learning/action plan

Case study 7.3

George Blow is a 52-year-old man with squamous cell carcinoma of the lung and bone metastases. He has recently completed a course of radiotherapy for symptom control. The district nursing team has been visiting to monitor and treat his skin reaction and to monitor his general condition. Today, his wife greets you at the door telling you 'George seems really muddled today and he hasn't eaten or drunk anything since yesterday because he says he feels nauseous'. You discuss with Mr Blow and his wife the importance of drinking enough fluids, and suggest he take his anti-emetic medication more regularly. The following day there is no improvement and his confusion seems to be worsening.

This is just an example. Keep your task simple. You could choose three or four cycles of evidence to demonstrate your competence each year.

Stage 1: Select your aspirations for good practice

The excellent nurse:

- can recognise medical emergencies in palliative care
- keeps the patient or relative informed about what is happening and how it can be treated
- makes timely referrals to medical colleagues.

Stage 2: Set the standards for your outcomes

Outcomes might include:

- the way learning is applied
- a learnt skill
- a protocol
- a strategy that is implemented
- meeting recommended standards.

- There is a record of how the practice team learns from a mistake to minimise a recurrence.

- The primary healthcare team is aware of medical emergencies in palliative care and has evidence-based care management plans to treat the emergency.

Stage 3A: Identify your learning needs

- Undertake a significant event audit of Mr Blow's case with the team responsible for his terminal care.
- Reflect on your knowledge of palliative care emergencies.
- Elicit views from patients/relatives/carers on how informed they felt about what was happening and their treatment.

Stage 3B: Identify your service needs

> Any of the needs assessment exercises in 3A may also reveal service needs.

- Invite a palliative care specialist (nurse or consultant) to talk to a meeting arranged for practices in your PCO to identify those conditions that are medical emergencies in palliative care, to improve recognition and treatment.
- Identify what resources are available in the practice for keeping the primary healthcare team up to date.

Stage 4: Make and carry out a learning and action plan

- Read up about palliative care emergencies and make a resource file so that other team members can refer to it.
- Work with the practice team to learn from the significant event audit of Mr Blow's case and make an action plan to minimise recurrence. You might develop care management plans for the treatment of palliative care emergencies.
- Attend and record learning points from the talk given by the palliative care specialist.

Stage 5: Document your learning, competence, performance and standards of service delivery

- Keep notes of the significant event audit and subsequent action plan.
- Include a copy of the audit of patient/relative/carer views on how informed they felt. Repeat the exercise after implementation of the action plan.
- Include a list of the learning points from the talk given by the palliative care specialist.
- Include a copy of the resource file on palliative care emergencies and care management plans that are available on the practice computer or in the practice library.

Case study 7.3 continued

You recognise that Mr Blow's symptoms may indicate hypercalcaemia and you contact the GP immediately to agree on blood tests required and the best course of action. Blood tests revealed dehydration and hypercalcaemia. Mr Blow is admitted for intravenous hydration and intravenous zoledronic acid 4 mg. On his return home he thanks you for taking such quick action. You continue to visit every two weeks to take blood to monitor his calcium levels and to assess his general condition and support both Mr Blow and his wife.

Example cycle of evidence 7.3

- Focus: communication
- Other relevant foci: working with colleagues; maintaining good nursing practice

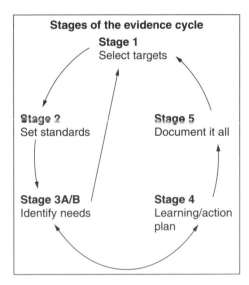

Stages of the evidence cycle

Stage 1
Select targets

Stage 2
Set standards

Stage 5
Document it all

Stage 3A/B
Identify needs

Stage 4
Learning/action plan

Case study 7.4

Mrs L is in the terminal phase from breast cancer and is receiving end-of-life care from the district nurses and the GP as she has requested to remain at home. When you visit this morning, her husband tells you she has had a 'bad night' and they had to call out the out-of-hours service to deal with her increased pain and restlessness. They had had to go through her whole history and all the medication she was on with the doctor who came, but in the end he gave her an injection and left a note requesting you to increase the diamorphine dosage and add midazolam to the medication in her syringe driver.

This is just an example. Keep your task simple. You could choose three or four cycles of evidence to demonstrate your competence each year.

Stage 1: Select your aspirations for good practice

The excellent nurse:

- ensures information is communicated within the team and other professionals as appropriate
- plans ahead to reduce the need for crisis management
- regularly updates information given to out-of-hours services to ensure continuity of care
- cares appropriately for patients in the last days of life.

Stage 2: Set the standards for your outcomes

Outcomes might include:

- the way learning is applied
- a learnt skill
- a protocol
- a strategy that is implemented
- meeting recommended standards.

- A system is in place for transferring and acting on information about patients seen by other nurses or doctors out of hours.
- Agreed plans for end-of-life care are initiated when patients enter the terminal phase of their illness.

Stage 3A: Identify your learning needs

- Audit via a retrospective case note analysis of ten patients with terminal cancer, to help you identify which aspects of care had not been planned and required crisis management.
- Obtain feedback from out-of-hours nursing services to assess the quality of the information communicated in relation to patients in the terminal phase, and the extent to which the information is regularly updated.
- Compare your practice against nationally recognised care of the dying pathway, such as the care pathway in the GSF.[2]

Stage 3B: Identify your service needs

> Any of the needs assessment exercises in 3A may also reveal service needs.

- Self-assess your primary healthcare team practice in the provision of cancer services using the 'good practice' self assessment tool.[13]
- Review the arrangements within the practice for transfer of information between team members and out-of-hours services for terminal care.

Stage 4: Make and carry out a learning and action plan

- Attend a GSF workshop.
- Nominate a co-ordinator for palliative care within the practice.
- Reflect on the feedback from the out-of-hours nursing service on communicating information about patients in the terminal phase, and develop a system, for example using a handover form.
- Reflect on the outcome of the self-assessment tool with the primary healthcare team. Make a plan to improve the provision of service for cancer care, and discuss adopting and using the care pathways.
- Obtain advice from the primary care organisation, from the primary care cancer lead, about how to improve communication and continuity of care and how to implement the GSF within your practice

Stage 5: Document your learning, competence, performance and standards of service delivery

- Keep a record of your discussion with the primary care cancer lead and document your plans for agreeing and implementing the GSF.
- Keep a copy of the last days of life care pathway.
- Record the outcome of the self-assessment tool.
- Keep a record of your notes on what you learnt on the GSF workshop with your certificate of attendance.
- Record how the system for communicating information with the out-of-hours services will be set up and used, and keep a copy of the handover form.

Case study 7.4 continued

You start Mrs L on the 'last days of life care pathway' and you fax the completed handover form to the out-of-hours nursing and medical services and the out-of-hours deputising service. All the discussion with the practice team and the PCO has been worthwhile in improving the care of patients with cancer, and the practice team is pleased with the improved lines of communication and the continuity of care for their patients, as well as ensuring that the practice can justify claiming the quality points for cancer care.

References

1 www.ncpc.org.uk

2 NHS Modernisation Agency (2003) *Gold Standards Framework Project in Community Palliative Care.* Department of Health, London. www.modern.nhs.uk/cancer (accessed 29 April 2005)

3 www.nice.org.uk (accessed 29 April 2005)

4 Macmillan Cancer Relief Fund: www.macmillan.org.uk (accessed 29 April 2005) Telephone helpline: freephone +44 (0)808 808 2020; textphone +44 (0)808 808 0121 Monday to Friday 9 am–6 pm.

5 Joint Formulary Committee (2005) *British National Formulary.* British Medical Association/Royal Pharmaceutical Society, London. www.bnf.org (accessed 29 April 2005)

6 Fallon M and O'Neill B (eds) (1998) *ABC of Palliative Care.* BMJ Books, London.

7 Twycross R, Wilcock A, Charlesworth S and Dickman A (2002) *Palliative Care Formulary (PCF2)* (2e). Radcliffe Medical Press Ltd, Oxford.

8 Tavares M (2003) *National Guidelines for the Use of Complementary Therapy.* The Prince of Wales's Foundation for Integrated Health London, England. www.hospice-spc-council.org.uk/public/complementaryguidelines.pdf

9 Ernst E (2000) Herbal medicine: where is the evidence? *British Medical Journal.* **321**: 395–6.

10 Medicines Control Agency (2002) *Safety of Herbal Medicinal Products.* Department of Health, London. www.mca.gov.uk/ourwork/licensingmeds/herbalmeds/HerbalsSafetyReportJuly2002_Final.pdf (accessed 29 April 2005)

11 Fallowfield L and Jenkins V (2004) Communicating sad, bad and difficult news in medicine. *The Lancet.* **363**: 312–19.

12 www.ovacome.org.uk (accessed 29 April 2005)

13 NHS Modernisation Agency (2004) *Cancer in Primary Care: a guide to good practice.* Modernisation Agency, London. www.modern.nhs.uk/cancer/primarycare (accessed 29 April 2005)

8

Osteoporosis

Nurses frequently take a lead role in the management of chronic diseases or long-term conditions. Please reread the introduction to Chapter 4 about your need to be qualified for a specialist role or that of community matron.

Osteoporosis is a disorder characterised by compromised bone strength. This bone disease is very common and many nurses, particularly those working with older people, are likely to encounter patients with it. The main consequence of osteoporosis is the increased tendency to fracture with minor trauma and the subsequent loss of function and quality of life. Colles' fracture affects 15% of women and vertebral fractures up to 20% (although many are asymptomatic). Hip fracture affects one in four of women who live to 85 years, a quarter of whom die within 12 months and more than half remain disabled.[1]

Case study 8.1

You are surprised to see Mrs Gaunt, a 52-year-old woman, as she rarely consults for herself. Her husband has been on long-term sickness benefit and she works long hours as a caretaker at a local school. She tells you stiffly that her mother has just died aged 68 years, following a fall in the house when she broke her hip. The specialist at the hospital told her that her mother's bones had crumbled away and that she and her younger sister should have a bone scan.

What issues you should cover

Although the family history is one indicator of risk, you will want to find out how many risk factors Mrs Gaunt might have. For example:

- being female: females have an increased risk
- being elderly: she is not that yet
- early menopause: ask about when her periods stopped
- smoking: ask about previous and current use
- high alcohol intake: mainly because of decreased nutrition
- physical inactivity: this is unlikely given her employment
- thin body type: this you can observe
- heredity: establish if her mother had any particular risk factors that might not be inherited, such as one of the secondary causes in Box 8.1
- secondary osteoporosis (*see* Box 8.1).

Box 8.1:   Types of osteoporosis

Primary

- Type 1 (postmenopausal)
- Type 2 (age-related bone loss)
- Idiopathic (at ages less than 50 years)

Secondary

- Endocrine e.g. thyrotoxicosis, primary hyperparathyroidism, Cushing's syndrome
- Hypogonadism, from anorexia nervosa or excessive exercise
- Gastrointestinal e.g. malabsorption such as coeliac disease, partial gastrectomy, liver disease
- Rheumatological e.g. rheumatoid arthritis, ankylosing spondylitis
- Malignancy e.g. multiple myeloma, metastases
- Drugs e.g. corticosteroids, heparin

Bone scan investigations

Dual energy x-ray absorptiometry (DXA) is the most widely used method of measuring bone mineral density (BMD). Using DXA confirms the diagnosis of osteoporosis, contributes to the assessment of risk of future fractures, and allows the most appropriate targeting of treatments.

Currently there is no rationale for population screening for low bone density. It makes sense to target those most likely to be at risk from the above lists. You might investigate a perimenopausal woman who has risk factors, to help her make a decision about using hormone replacement therapy. Similarly, you might wish to screen younger women with risk factors such as premature menopause or anorexia nervosa. Other indications would be those patients with diseases causing secondary osteoporosis (*see* Box 8.1), patients on more than 7.5 mg prednisolone or equivalent for more than 6 months, or those with a low impact fracture. Your local bone density screening unit is likely to have a list of criteria that Mrs Gaunt must satisfy before she can be screened, and it would be helpful to go through these with her to determine how much at risk she is.

Results of bone density scans

If osteoporosis (T score −1 to −2.5) or osteopenia (T score below −2.5) is found, you should screen for underlying causes with other investigations:

- serum calcium, phosphate, alkaline phosphatase, and creatinine
- serum protein electrophoresis
- thyroid function tests
- serum testosterone in men

- urinary Bence–Jones protein, or 24 hour urinary calcium or creatinine excretion as indicated by the clinical findings and consultation with the laboratory.

Treatment for those patients with osteopenia or osteoporosis

You would want to ensure that all patients at risk receive lifestyle advice, i.e. regular weight-bearing exercise, adequate nutrition including calcium and vitamin D, and avoidance of smoking or excess alcohol. Preventing falls minimises fracture risk and a useful summary of strategies appears in the *Drug and Therapeutics Bulletin* on managing falls in older people,[2] and in the National Institute for Clinical Excellence (NICE) guideline on the *Assessment and Prevention of Falls in Older People.*[3] You will want to minimise other risk factors, but this may not be possible, e.g. for a patient needing steroid treatment. An understanding of the guidelines for the prevention and treatment of glucocorticoid-induced osteoporosis is important for nurse prescribers who wish to develop their competency in this area of care.[4] Education about osteoporosis for patients, carers and relatives is very helpful, and the National Osteoporosis Society produces relevant material as well as a patient helpline and an email address for nursing queries.[5]

Pain relief for established osteoporosis is mainly by analgesic medication working up from paracetamol in full dosage to opiates. Remember that opiates or opiate-like drugs may increase the risk of falling. Low-dose antidepressants are useful for their pain-modulating effects and you might wish to refer to the pain clinic. Lumbar supports, transcutaneous nerve stimulators, or acupuncture are useful.

Non-pharmacological interventions shown to have positive effects on bone density in men and postmenopausal women include:[6]

- exercise programmes combining low impact weight-bearing exercise and high-intensity strength training (high-impact training e.g. jumping is not suitable for patients with osteoporosis)
- diet-derived calcium intake of 1000 mg calcium per day.

Drug treatments for improving bone mass (or preventing further loss) are summarised in the guidelines from the Royal College of Physicians,[7] and the medications in Box 8.2 should be considered for established osteoporosis or for osteopenia with a history of previous fracture. NICE has also published guidelines covering the treatment of secondary prevention of osteoporotic fragility fractures in postmenopausal women who have sustained an osteoporotic fracture.[8]

Table 8.1: Drugs to improve bone mass[1,7,9]

Drug	Guidelines
Vitamin D and calcium	Recommended daily dose 800 IU of vitamin D and 0.5–1 g of calcium. Has been shown to reduce hip fracture in frail elderly, modest reduction in non-vertebral fracture in men and women over 65 years. Usually used as adjuncts to other treatments
Calcium	At 1000 mg daily has a less marked effect than when given with vitamin D
Calcitriol, ergocalciferol, alphacalcidol	These vitamin D supplements given at pharmacological dosage require plasma calcium monitoring
Biphosphonates e.g. aledronate, etidronate, risenronate	Poor absorption means they should be taken on an empty stomach, but they can cause gastrointestinal problems. Once weekly dosage now available
Hormone replacement therapy e.g. oestrogen, testosterone	Treatment should be for at least five years to decrease the fracture risk, long-term treatment risks (e.g. increased cancer breast or prostate) must be balanced against gains
Selective oestrogen receptor modulators (SERMS) e.g. raloxifene	SERMs like raloxifene are useful for those women who do not require relief of hot flushes, or who need to avoid the oestrogen-stimulating effect on the endometrium or breast
Calcitonin or teriparatide	Available as subcutaneous injection; it also has analgesic effects useful in acute fracture
Anabolic steroids	Androgenic side-effects make these unsuitable for women

Collecting data to demonstrate your learning, competence, performance and standards of service delivery

Example cycle of evidence 8.1

- Focus: complaints
- Other relevant foci: working with colleagues; teaching and training; relationships with patients

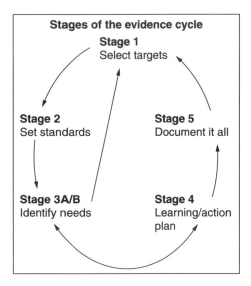

Stages of the evidence cycle

Stage 1
Select targets

Stage 2
Set standards

Stage 5
Document it all

Stage 3A/B
Identify needs

Stage 4
Learning/action plan

Case study 8.2

Your practice has received a patient complaint about you, the practice nurse who leads on family planning. Mrs Prog is concerned that her daughter Sarah is on Depo-Provera contraceptive injections which she has read on the internet has an adverse effect on bones and may lead to osteoporosis, and that the practice has not offered her an alternative contraception method.

This is just an example. Keep your task simple. You could choose three or four cycles of evidence to demonstrate your competence each year.

Stage 1: Select your aspirations for good practice

The excellent nurse:

- apologises appropriately when things go wrong, and has an adequate complaints procedure in place
- makes sure that she has access to all updated information and guidance from the Medicines and Healthcare products Regulatory Agency (MHRA).[10]

Stage 2: Set the standards for your outcomes

Outcomes might include:

- the way learning is applied
- a learnt skill
- a protocol
- a strategy that is implemented
- meeting recommended standards.

- Understand and establish effective processes for preventing and managing complaints from patients in the practice.
- Ensure that health professionals have adequate opportunities for keeping up to date.

Stage 3A: Identify your learning needs

- Examine as a significant event one or more complaints, e.g. where the practice has not advised a patient correctly about the complaints process.
- Compare the actual care of the patient against an acceptable standard of care for patients with risk of osteoporosis. Use peer review by asking respected colleagues, such as the osteoporosis nurse specialist in your area, or compare your practice against a published standard such as a guideline by a responsible body of professional opinion.[6]
- Review the way that you obtain supervision and appraisal and how your personal and professional development plan is being implemented.

Stage 3B: Identify your service needs

Any of the needs assessment exercises in 3A may also reveal service needs.

- Audit patient complaints in the preceding 12 months: the number, the outcomes and how the complaint system is advertised, etc.

- Audit the extent to which doctors and nurses are following practice-agreed protocols. This is about being proactive about preventing or minimising the likelihood of the source of the complaint recurring.
- Audit vulnerable areas. Look back at the analysis of complaints to identify useful areas for focusing learning, e.g. a review the use of bone-protective agents in people prescribed oral steroids.

Stage 4: Make and carry out a learning and action plan

- Ask your primary care organisation to look at the practice complaints system and feed back on how it can be improved (if at all).
- Arrange a tutorial between the practice manager and others in the team about preventing and managing complaints, or use one of the risk management packages produced by medical defence organisations.[11,12]
- Read up on how to undertake significant event analysis, including how to share the information with the practice team and respond as a practice team.
- Find out how to add a reminder to the records of patients at risk of osteoporosis.

Stage 5: Document your learning, competence, performance and standards of service delivery

- Keep a copy of how the complaint was managed.
- Produce a protocol of the patient complaint process against which consecutive complaints can be audited in another 12 months' time.
- Keep a record of how you will assess clinical supervision and how you will be helped, following appraisal with your personal and professional development plan.
- Record how you added a reminder to the records of patients with risk factors for osteoporosis.

Case study 8.2 continued

Mrs Prog and her daughter Sarah meet with the practice manager, the GP and yourself. During the discussion, it becomes apparent that Sarah blames herself for finding it difficult to remember a daily pill, while Mrs Prog is angry that her daughter had not been aware of the possible adverse effects. Since the complaint, Sarah has been offered an alternative contraception method. The practice manager says she will ensure all MHRA advice and guidance will be forwarded to you via email. You rearrange regular supervision meetings with the GP who has the lead for family planning that had been allowed to lapse due to pressure of work.

Example cycle of evidence 8.2

- Focus: keeping good records
- Other relevant foci: maintaining good nursing practice; prescribing; working with colleagues

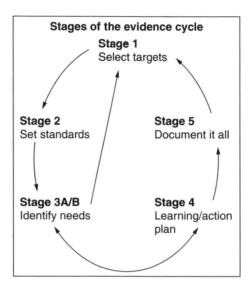

Stages of the evidence cycle

Stage 1
Select targets

Stage 2
Set standards

Stage 5
Document it all

Stage 3A/B
Identify needs

Stage 4
Learning/action plan

Case study 8.3

Mrs Dirge is not a welcome name on your patient list. She consults frequently but has so many things wrong with her that it is difficult to know how to manage any one complaint. She has hypertension, diabetes, chronic obstructive airways disease, osteoarthritis and has recently developed polymyalgia rheumatica, and was prescribed high-dose steroids. She usually consults your colleague who has been on sick leave for two months and you feel a momentary irritation that here is another burden for those left to cope. Among several other complaints, she wants something for indigestion and says she could not take the tablets the GP had recently given her. Looking at her recent prescription list, you see that she has had several different antacid medications repeated, two different proton pump inhibitors, is still taking naproxen as well as prednisolone and has stopped the Didronel PMO pack (disodium etidronate and calcium carbonate).

This is just an example. Keep your task simple. You could choose three or four cycles of evidence to demonstrate your competence each year.

Stage 1: Select your aspirations for good practice

The excellent nurse:

- makes sound management decisions which are based on good practice and evidence, supported by a comprehensive clinical management plan (CMP)
- records appropriate information for all contacts
- only prescribes treatments that make an effective contribution to the patient's overall management and which are listed on the agreed CMP.

Stage 2: Set the standards for your outcomes

Outcomes might include:

- the way learning is applied
- a learnt skill
- a protocol
- a strategy that is implemented
- meeting recommended standards.

- The practice has an effective repeat prescribing policy that is consistently applied.
- The practice has an agreed policy for managing the needs of patients when the usual health professional responsible is absent.

Stage 3A: Identify your learning needs

- Note in your reflective diary your concerns about the repeat prescribing, the lack of overall control and the inappropriate use of antacids.
- Obtain feedback from ten patients who usually see your absent colleague about how their needs are being managed, to determine whether your irritation and overwork (and that of others in the practice) is affecting their care.

Stage 3B: Identify your service needs

Any of the needs assessment exercises in 3A may also reveal service needs.

- Arrange for an anonymous comment form about repeat prescribing and how it works in practice to be completed by staff members involved.
- Conduct a SWOT analysis of repeat prescribing by the practice team, with a subsequent action plan to update or revise current practice policy.
- Arrange an audit of the adherence of the practice team to the repeat prescribing policy.
- Identify whether more health professional time is needed to manage patient need.

Stage 4: Make and carry out a learning and action plan

- Meet up with a pharmaceutical advisor to discuss repeat prescribing policy and the prescribing of antacids, gastroprotection for patients on steroids and NSAIDs and the best use of biphosphonates for bone protection. Meet the advisor on your own or with practice colleagues.
- Attend a workshop on the management of multiple medication.
- Discuss the audit and/or SWOT analysis results, proposed revisions to practice repeat prescribing in general, and the suggestions from the prescribing advisor to agree revisions to the practice protocol for repeat prescribing.

Stage 5: Document your learning, competence, performance and standards of service delivery

- Keep extracts from your reflective diary about the difficulties and the changes made to remedy them.
- Record the actions to increase health professional time available to manage patient need.
- Include the results of the audit, SWOT analysis and notes from the meeting with the prescribing advisor and the action plan that followed.
- Include a copy of the revised repeat prescribing policy.

Case study 8.3 continued

You explain briefly to Mrs Dirge that her medication is upsetting her stomach but that some of it is essential. You give her the repeat prescription slip with one of the proton pump inhibitors highlighted, and ask her to take that very regularly to protect her stomach. You ask her to fill a carrier bag with all the medication she has been given and bring it to another (longer) appointment with her to go through it all and rationalise it. You make a note to go through her records and make sure that she is not taking anything that she does not have to take in order to reduce the risk of iatrogenic symptoms.

Example cycle of evidence 8.3

- Focus: evidence-based care
- Other relevant focus: clinical care

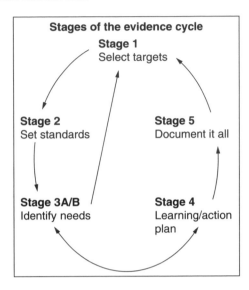

Stages of the evidence cycle

Stage 1
Select targets

Stage 2
Set standards

Stage 5
Document it all

Stage 3A/B
Identify needs

Stage 4
Learning/action plan

Case study 8.4

Mrs Menses attends for her annual review of hormone replacement therapy (HRT) treatment. You see in her records that she has been on HRT for 5 years now for menopausal symptoms. Following discussion about benefits and potential risks, Mrs Menses decides to stop HRT and you explain that she should phase it out slowly. After Mrs Menses has left, you consider the implications of her stopping HRT in relation to her risk of osteoporosis, which is particularly common in postmenopausal women.

This is just an example. Keep your task simple. You could choose three or four cycles of evidence to demonstrate your competence each year.

Stage 1: Select your aspirations for good practice

The excellent nurse:

- is aware of the risk factors for osteoporosis
- knows how to refer for bone density scanning
- has a basic knowledge of treatments for osteoporosis and can explain them to patients
- is aware of local services for ostcoporosis.

Stage 2: Set the standards for your outcomes

Outcomes might include:

- the way learning is applied
- a learnt skill
- a protocol
- a strategy that is implemented
- meeting recommended standards.

- The practice has a protocol on screening for osteoporosis.
- The practice has library and patient literature on osteoporosis.

Stage 3A: Identify your learning needs

- Find out if paper based resources (e.g. books or files) or electronic sites describing best practice in management of osteoporosis are easily accessed by you in your practice.
- Reflect on whether you are up to date with current treatments for osteoporosis.
- Review what services are available locally for osteoporosis.

Stage 3B: Identify your service needs

Any of the needs assessment exercises in 3A may also reveal service needs.

- Compare best practice in the management of osteoporosis with the practice protocol if available and update as required.
- Audit the waiting time for DXA screening in your locality by reviewing the length of time waited by the previous 20 patients referred for bone density scan, or by discussing with the PCO commissioning lead.
- Review what literature is available to patients in the practice in relation to osteoporosis, and ask several patients to comment on the patient information leaflet to check that it is suitable for patients in your population.

Stage 4: Make and carry out a learning and action plan

- Meet up with PCO commissioning lead to discuss waiting times for bone density scanning.
- Write out what constitutes best practice in investigating patients at risk of osteoporosis and the treatment of osteoporosis. Then agree a practice template for screening with the primary healthcare team.
- Spend time or have a tutorial with the osteoporosis nurse specialist in your area to increase your knowledge of local services.
- Compile a list of library or other resources (paper/electronic) your practice needs to buy so that there is sufficient reference material available in relation to osteoporosis. Check your choice with the local health librarian if possible and place an order.

Stage 5: Document your learning, competence, performance and standards of service delivery

- Keep a copy of the practice template and protocol on the screening and management of osteoporosis.
- List the contents of the reference library in the practice and the resources available in each consulting room including patient information leaflets.[3]
- Keep a record of the notes made at your visit to the osteoporosis nurse specialist.
- Record the discussion with the PCO on waiting times for bone density scanning and the PCO's plans to improve access.

Case study 8.4 continued

You see Mrs Menses at a follow-up visit and review her risk factors for osteoporosis. You complete the screening template and give her lifestyle advice and arrange for her referral for DXA scan. You give her the patient information leaflets to support the verbal advice you have already given. The practice team is pleased to know that their management of osteoporosis is based on up-to-date evidence.

References

1 Snaith ML (ed.) (1999) *ABC of Rheumatology*. BMJ Books, London.

2 Drugs and Therapeutics Bulletin (2000) Managing falls in older people. *Drugs and Therapeutics Bulletin*. **38**: 68–72.

3 National Institute for Clinical Excellence (NICE) (2004) *Falls: the assessment and prevention of falls in older people*. NICE, London.

4 Royal College of Physicians, Bone and Tooth Society of Great Britain, National Osteoporosis Society (2002) *Glucocorticoid-Induced Osteoporosis: guidelines for prevention and treatment*. Royal College of Physicians, London.

5   National Osteoporosis Society, PO Box 10, Radstock, Bath BA3 3YB, UK. Patient helpline tel: +44 (0)1761 472721. www.nos.org.uk (accessed 29 April 2005). For nursing queries email: nurses@nos.org.uk

6   Scottish Intercollegiate Guidelines Network (SIGN) (2003) *Management of Osteoporosis – a national clinical guideline.* SIGN, Edinburgh. www.sign.ac.uk (accessed 29 April 2005)

7   Royal College of Physicians, Bone and Tooth Society of Great Britain (2000) *Osteoporosis. Clinical guidelines for prevention and treatment. Update of pharmacological interventions and an algorithm for management.* Royal College of Physicians of London, London.

8   National Institute for Clinical Excellence (NICE) (2005) Bisphosphonates, selective oestrogen receptor modulators and parathyroid hormone for the secondary prevention of osteoporotic fragility fractures in postmenopausal women. NICE, London. www.nice.org.uk (accessed 29 April 2005)

9   Compston J (2000) Updated guidelines on osteoporosis include management algorithm. *Guidelines in Practice.* **3**: 23–8.

10 Medicines and Healthcare products Regulatory Agency website: www.mhra.gov.uk (accessed 29 April 2005)

11 MPS Risk Consulting, Granary Wharf House, Leeds LS11 5PY, UK. www.mps-riskconsulting.com (accessed 29 April 2005)

12 MDU Services Ltd, 230 Blackfriars Road, London SE1 8PJ, UK. www.the-mdu.com (accessed 29 April 2005)

And finally

We hope that you have found that the stages in our 'cycle of evidence' are a useful approach to gathering information about what you need to learn. You can also use it to identify improvements you or others need to make to the way you deliver services.

It is easy to feel overwhelmed by the magnitude of the task to demonstrate that you are competent and perform consistently well as a nurse, in order to retain your registration to practise. Remember, in order to re-register with the NMC, you should be producing evidence about the breadth of your practice, every three years. Take your time and select three or four cycles of evidence each year. Try to get into the habit of reflective writing to learn from critical incidents, and include these in your portfolio. Recognise that you have achieved change in practice and remember to put the documentary evidence on your portfolio. Use the portfolio as a teaching aid with students and junior staff to show that the process of lifelong learning is a reality.

Ask others for help. Your line manager, colleagues and practice staff should be able to help you to collect information about what you need to learn, or about gaps in services. You may be able to use information that has been already collected or you may be able to delegate some of the administrative side. Your colleagues or your patients will be well placed to help you to set your aspirations for good practice and set achievable standards for your outcomes – of learning and improvements in service delivery. Perhaps at your appraisal you can develop learning and action in your PDP. These cycles of evidence will be the nucleus of your PDP. Colleagues in the team can support you in documenting the evidence of your competence, performance and subsequent standards of service delivery. Other books in this series might help you to look at specific clinical areas, especially those where quality frameworks or special interests require your attention. Remember to visit this book's supporting website, which includes useful website links.[1]

So the evidence will be there ready to submit for appraisal, re-registration, prescribing competency or when applying for a new job, but the results will show what a good nurse you really are. The patients you care for will be the ones to benefit most from your efforts to provide optimal quality. This should give you increasing confidence and self-respect. Enjoy your professional glow.

Reference

1 http://health.mattersonline.net

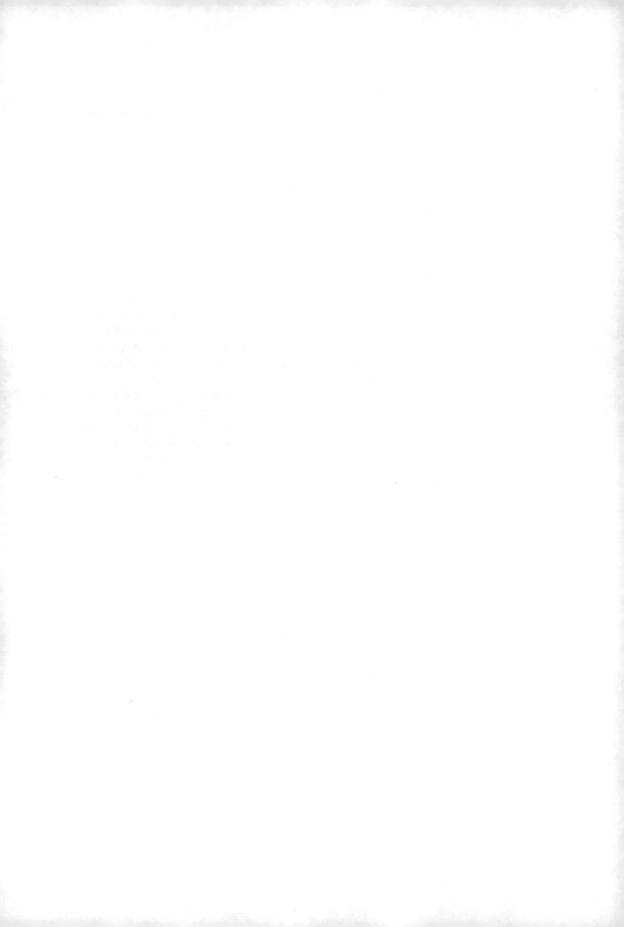

INDEX